ABC OF
RHEUMATOLOGY

Third Edition

ABC OF
RHEUMATOLOGY

Third Edition

Edited by

MICHAEL L SNAITH MD FRCP
Senior Lecturer in Rheumatology, University of Sheffield
and
Honorary Consultant Rheumatologist, Royal Hallamshire Hospital, Sheffield

BMJ
Books

First edition 1986
Second edition 1999
Third edition 2004
by BMJ Publishing Group Ltd., BMA House, Tavistock Square,
London WC1H 9JR

www.bmjbooks.com

British Library Cataloguing in Publication Data

A catalogue record for this book is available from the British Library

ISBN 0 7279 1688 2

Typeset by Newgen Imaging Systems (P) Ltd., Chennai, India
Printed and bound in Spain by Graphycems, Navarra

The cover shows a fluorescent anti-DNA antibody test. The substrate (target) is *Crithidia lucilae*—showing specific antibody to double-stranded DNA in a patient with systemic lupus erythematosus

Contents

	Contributors	*vi*
	Preface	*vii*
	Acknowledgments	*viii*
1	**Community rheumatology: delivering care across boundaries** *Elaine M Hay*	1
2	**Pain in the wrist and hand** *Michael A Shipley*	4
3	**Pain in the neck, shoulder, and upper arm** *Cathy Speed*	10
4	**Low back pain** *Cathy Speed*	15
5	**Pain in the hip and knee** *Andrew J Hamer*	19
6	**Pain in the foot** *James Woodburn, Philip S Helliwell*	23
7	**Fibromyalgia: musculoskeletal distress** *Sarah Ryan, Anne Browne*	30
8	**Osteoarthritis** *Nicholas Raj, Adrian Jones*	34
9	**Gout and hyperuricaemia** *Michael L Snaith, Adewale O Adebajo*	39
10	**Osteoporosis** *Nicola Peel, Richard Eastell*	45
11	**Rheumatoid arthritis: clinical features and diagnosis** *Mohammed Akil, Kiran Veerapen*	50
12	**Rheumatoid arthritis: treatment** *Mohammed Akil, Kiran Veerapen*	56
13	**Spondyloarthropathies** *Gabrielle Kingsley, Non Pugh*	61
14	**Juvenile idiopathic arthritis** *Mark Friswell, Tauny R Southwood*	68
15	**Polymyalgia rheumatica and giant cell arteritis** *Maya H Buch, Howard A Bird*	75
16	**Systemic lupus erythematosus, antiphospholipid antibody syndrome, and other lupus-like syndromes** *Tsui-Yee Lian, Caroline Gordon*	80
17	**Raynaud's phenomenon and scleroderma** *Christopher P Denton, Carol M Black*	87
18	**Is it a connective tissue disease?** *Peter J Maddison*	92
19	**Vasculitis and related rashes** *Richard A Watts, David GI Scott*	98
20	**Laboratory tests** *Margaret J Larché, David A Isenberg*	103
21	**The team approach** *Janet Cushnaghan, Jackie McDowell*	110
22	**Epidemiology of rheumatic diseases** *Alex J MacGregor, Timothy D Spector*	114
	Index	121

Contributors

Adewale O Adebajo
Consultant Rheumatologist, Barnsley District General Hospital, Barnsley, Yorkshire

Mohammed Akil
Consultant Rheumatologist, Royal Hallamshire Hospital, Sheffield

Howard A Bird
Professor of Pharmacological Rheumatology, Chapel Allerton Hospital, Leeds

Carol M Black
Professor of Rheumatology and Centre Director, Royal Free Hospital, London

Anne Browne
Nurse Consultant in Rheumatology, Pennine Acute Hospitals NHS Trust, Royal Oldham Hospital, Oldham

Maya H Buch
ARC Research Fellow and Specialist Registrar, Academic Unit of Musculoskeletal Disease, Leeds General Infirmary

Janet Cushnaghan
Rheumatology Practitioner, Lymington Hospital, Hampshire

Christopher P Denton
Senior Lecturer and Consultant Rheumatologist, Centre for Rheumatology, Royal Free Hospital, London

Richard Eastell
Professor of Bone Metabolism, Division of Clinical Sciences, Northern General Hospital, Sheffield

Mark Friswell
Consultant Paediatric Rheumatologist, Freeman Hospital, Newcastle-upon-Tyne

Caroline Gordon
Reader and Consultant in Rheumatology, Department of Rheumatology, The Medical School, University of Birmingham

Andrew J Hamer
Consultant Orthopaedic Surgeon, Northern General Hospital, Sheffield

Elaine M Hay
Professor of Community Rheumatology, University Hospital of North Staffordshire NHS Trust

Philip S Helliwell
Senior Lecturer in Rheumatology, Academic Unit of Musculoskeletal Disease, University of Leeds

David A Isenberg
ARC Diamond Professor of Rheumatology, University College London Hospitals

Adrian Jones
Consultant Rheumatologist, Nottingham City Hospital, Nottingham

Gabrielle Kingsley
Reader in Rheumatology, Guy's, King's and St Thomas's School of Medicine, London and Consultant Rheumatologist, University Hospital, Lewisham, London

Margaret J Larché
Clinical Research Fellow, Kennedy Institute of Rheumatology, London

Tsui-Yee Lian
Staff Rheumatologist, Rheumatology, Allergy and Immunology Department, Tan Tock Seng Hospital, Singapore

Alex J MacGregor
Professor of Chronic Disease Epidemiology and Honorary Consultant Rheumatologist, School of Medicine, Health Policy and Practice, University of East Anglia, Norwich

Peter J Maddison
Consultant Rheumatologist, North West Wales NHS Trust and Professor of Joint and Muscle Disorders, School of Sport, Health and Exercise Sciences, University of Wales, Bangor

Jackie McDowell
Rheumatology Clinical Specialist, County Hospital, Hereford

Nicola Peel
Consultant in Metabolic Bone Medicine, Metabolic Bone Centre, Sheffield Teaching Hospitals NHS Trust

Non Pugh
Consultant Rheumatologist, Gwent NHS Healthcare Trust, Wales

Nicholas Raj
Specialist Registrar, Rheumatology Department, Nottingham City Hospital

Sarah Ryan
Nurse Consultant in Rheumatology, Staffordshire Rheumatology Centre, University Hospital of North Staffordshire

David GI Scott
Consultant Rheumatologist, Norfolk and Norwich University Hospital NHS Trust, and Honorary Professor, University of East Anglia

Michael A Shipley
Consultant Rheumatologist, University College London Hospitals

Michael L Snaith
Senior Lecturer in Rheumatology, University of Sheffield and Honorary Consultant Rheumatologist, Royal Hallamshire Hospital, Sheffield

Tauny R Southwood
Professor of Paediatric Rheumatology, University of Birmingham

Timothy D Spector
Consultant Rheumatologist, St Thomas's Hospital and Professor of Genetic Epidemiology, St George's Hospital, London

Cathy Speed
Honorary Consultant, Rheumatology and Sports Medicine, Addenbrooke's Hospital, Cambridge

Kiran Veerapen
Consultant Rheumatologist, Division of Musculoskeletal Sciences, Sunway Medical Centre, Petaling Jaya, Malaysia

Richard A Watts
Consultant Rheumatologist, Ipswich Hospital NHS Trust

James Woodburn
MRC Clinician Scientist Fellow and Honorary Podiatrist, Academic Unit of Musculoskeletal Disease, University of Leeds

Preface

We have considerably revised the *ABC of Rheumatology* for the third edition. There are two new chapters on community rheumatology and "Is it a connective tissue disease?" All existing chapters have new authors or co-authors. The style of presentation has been unified. Guidance for further reading has been revised, with references to useful reviews and, where appropriate, research literature. Nevertheless, the emphasis of the book remains clinical. The first section covers common regional musculoskeletal problems, followed by a greater focus on systemic disorders and pathology.

We considered a separate ABC for the rheumatic conditions seen in Africa, the Pacific Rim and Far East. However, it seemed to us that it would be more sensible to recognise that although there are some geographically distinct musculoskeletal disorders, in the main the differences are those of emphasis rather than pathology. Accordingly, I have recruited colleagues with knowledge of rheumatic conditions as seen in India, Africa, and Asia. They have co-written chapters with UK-based colleagues with, I believe, an insight that has further enhanced the book for UK and overseas readers alike. I am most grateful to all the contributors to the third edition.

Michael Snaith
Derbyshire
2003

Acknowledgments

I should like to acknowledge with gratitude the friendly and professional encouragement and help of the staff of BMJ Books: Eleanor Lines, ABC series Commissioning Editor, Sally Carter, ABC series Development Editor, Naomi Wilkinson, Project Editor, and Nathan Harris, Production Executive.

   I wish to record my grateful thanks to my colleague Dr Ade Adebajo, for his contributions and helpful advice; and to Professor Peter Maddison and Dr Bill Egner for providing excellent illustrations which have been used in the production of this edition.

1 Community rheumatology: delivering care across boundaries

Elaine M Hay

The ever increasing demand on acute hospitals to deliver emergency medicine, together with technological (but time consuming and expensive) advances, means that follow up of many chronic conditions has been taken out of the acute setting and, by default, has been delegated to primary care. Unfortunately, this shift has not always been mirrored by appropriate shifts in resources and skills. This chapter looks at new ways of working to try to ensure that patients with musculoskeletal conditions receive timely, appropriate treatments despite the limitations of restricted resources.

Shared care—how to make it work

With hospital services running at full (or over) capacity, one solution is the use of "shared care." A simple transfer of the workload from rheumatologists to general practitioners will not help, because primary care also is bursting at the seams. One way in which rheumatological expertise can be transferred to the community without increasing the burden in primary care involves development of the skills of healthcare professionals such as nurses, physiotherapists, and occupational therapists. They can work in extended roles at high levels of clinical practice and cross traditional professional boundaries. They can be involved in assessment (of the disease and psychosocial factors), follow up, and management of patients with musculoskeletal conditions and inflammatory arthritis. Their roles and responsibilities have been defined recently.[1]

Role of the specialist nurse

Specialist nurses can provide a link between primary care and secondary care by acting as channels of communication between patients, general practitioners, and hospital specialists. Such nurses have a holistic approach to the management of chronic musculoskeletal conditions and are well placed to have an overall view of patients' care, which often can be fragmented. One example of where specialist nurses can have a pivotal role is the monitoring of patients with inflammatory arthritis who are taking disease modifying antirheumatic drugs. An average general practitioner has perhaps only 10-20 patients with rheumatoid arthritis and they will be taking a variety of disease modifying antirheumatic drugs. This makes it difficult for any individual general practitioner to gain the expertise and confidence needed to monitor the effects of these potentially dangerous drugs. The British Society for Rheumatology has proposed guidelines on how to monitor the effects of such drugs,[2] which could be used to develop guidelines for shared care in which specialist nurses liaise with general practitioners.

Which patients need secondary care?

Waiting times for new rheumatology appointments vary widely and depend on local resources, and to some extent, on how

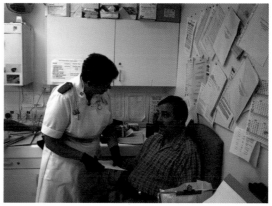

Specialist nurses can provide a link between primary and secondary care

---

Requirements for models of shared care
- Appropriate to local needs
- Responsive to local demands
- In the patients' best interests

Role of the specialist nurse
- Supervise treatment safety—for example, monitoring of disease modifying antirheumatic drugs
- Review treatment effectiveness
- Coordinate the multidisciplinary team
- Provide a communication channel between patients and the team
- Act as the patient's advocate
- Promote continuity of care
- Identify and address patients' psychosocial issues
- Facilitate education for patients, carers, and health professionals

---

doctors triage referrals from general practitioners. To make the system work effectively, care pathways need to make the patient a partner and take psychosocial as well as biomechanical factors into consideration. The outcome—in terms of whether the patient is given an appropriate level of priority with an appropriate healthcare professional—depends largely on the information given in the referral letter. Standardised referral forms may help, but they are time consuming to complete and rather impersonal.

Estimates show that 15% of all consultations with general practitioners are for musculoskeletal conditions. Most of these are for osteoarthritis in patients aged over 50 years and back pain in those under 50. One challenge for general practitioners is to spot among this caseload the small number of patients with early inflammatory arthritis, as they will benefit from early referral to hospital and prompt treatment with disease modifying antirheumatic drugs. No specific clinical, radiological, or immunological markers exist for rheumatoid arthritis. Normal blood test results and x ray results do not exclude rheumatoid arthritis, but equally a positive test for rheumatoid factor does not clinch the diagnosis. Most rheumatology departments promote an "inclusive approach" to referral and encourage general practitioners to be very suspicious and not to delay referral of patients with possible inflammatory arthritis. Ideally, patients who may have inflammatory problems will be fast tracked to secondary care.

Primary care management of musculoskeletal problems

Clearly, most patients who present to general practitioners will not have inflammatory arthritis. Indeed for many patients, a precise pathological diagnosis based on symptoms, signs, and results of investigations will not be possible and may not be the most appropriate approach to management. This "medical model" of care often fails to consider other important influences on pain perception, such as emotional and behavioural factors, and it may encourage chronicity by using terms such as "arthritis," "wear and tear," or "degeneration," which emphasise the unchanging nature of the condition. Doctors are trained to diagnose "disease," whereas the patient's concern is what to do about their musculoskeletal pain—not just what to call it.

An alternative approach, which may be more useful in primary care, limits the diagnostic process to identification of potentially serious pathologies or other specific diseases or disorders—the so called "red flag" disorders. This system was initially developed for back pain and has been effective in changing the management of this condition in primary care. It applies equally well to other widespread or regional pain disorders.[3] Broadly speaking, patients with "red flags" should be considered for referral to secondary care for further investigation and management.

After the small proportion of patients with potentially serious conditions have been excluded and dealt with, the general practitioner must then decide how best to manage the remaining patients. Two areas need to be considered—how to deal with the presenting pain and distress (discussed below) and how to prevent future disability. Guidelines for the management of low back pain highlight how important it is to identify factors that predict chronicity. Positive messages about likely recovery and lack of long-term harm that take particular account of psychosocial barriers to recovery ("yellow flags") are important. These principles have been described elsewhere.[4]

Important information needed in referral letters for rheumatology appointments

- Length of history
- Pattern of joint involvement
- Presence of joint swelling
- Presence of early morning stiffness
- Previous treatments and response
- Level of distress or disability
- Results of investigations
- Other relevant medical or psychosocial factors

Symptoms and signs suggestive of early inflammatory arthritis

- Symmetrical soft tissue swelling (synovitis) of wrists, metacarpophalangeal joints, or proximal interphalangeal joints, or all three
- Joint stiffness a significant problem—especially early in the morning for longer than 30 minutes
- Soft tissue swelling of any joints
- Good response to trial of non-steroidal anti-inflammatory drugs

---

Red flags for regional pain syndromes

- History of considerable trauma
    Fracture
    Major soft tissue injury
- Localised joint swelling or redness, or both
    Septic arthritis
    Inflammatory arthritis
    Haemarthrosis
- Unremitting night pain
    Malignancy
    Inflammation or infection
- Bony tenderness
    Fracture
    Malignancy
    Infection
- Systemic disturbance
- Substantial comorbidity

Psychosocial factors that predict chronicity

- Belief that:
    pain is due to progressive pathology
    pain represents harm or injury
    avoidance of activity will speed up recovery
- Tendency to social isolation
- Tendency to anxiety or depression
- Expectation that passive treatments will be more of more benefit than self-help programmes

Evidence based treatment in primary care for musculoskeletal problems

The shift in emphasis towards self-management of musculoskeletal problems means that the primary healthcare team is of central importance. A growing base of evidence supports the effectiveness of a number of simple primary care interventions for musculoskeletal problems.[5] Direct access to physiotherapy shortens waiting times and reduces the costs associated with treatment and is one way of getting patients to use exercise and self-management regimens. Such regimens have been shown to be beneficial for patients with a variety of regional and widespread musculoskeletal conditions, including osteoarthritis, back pain, fibromyalgia, and shoulder problems. Prescribed exercise need not be the province of physiotherapists only: waiting times to see physiotherapists often are excessively long, and many self-limiting musculoskeletal conditions can be managed with sensible exercise regimens undertaken outside the hospital setting. This has the advantage of promoting self-help and "demedicalising" common musculoskeletal problems. Arthritis Research Campaign publishes a wide range of patient information leaflets and booklets that are useful adjuncts to the advice and education given by healthcare professionals.

Local steroid injections are effective at reducing pain from soft tissue problems such as tennis elbow and shoulder problems in the short term, but they do not improve long-term outcome. They should be reserved for patients in whom pain restricts rehabilitation with the measures discussed above. Although the risks from local steroid injections are minimal, certain precautions need to be taken.

Non-steroidal anti-inflammatory drugs may be beneficial for the short-term treatment of osteoarthritis, but they have a worrying side effect profile in the patients most likely to be prescribed them (elderly women). Simple analgesics are the preferred option where possible.

Arthritis Research Campaign information leaflets and booklets can be obtained through:
Arthritis Research Campaign
Copeman House
St Mary's Court
St Mary's Gate
Chesterfield
Derbyshire
S41 7TD
www.arc.org.uk

Contraindications to local steroid injections

Absolute	*Relative*
• Suspected septic arthritis	• Poorly controlled diabetes mellitus
• Local skin disorders or sepsis	• Osteoporosis
• Active systemic infection	
• Prosthetic joint	

Conclusion

Over the last ten years, the thinking on how best to care for patients with rheumatological disorders has changed. For patients with inflammatory arthritis, the emphasis is on prompt referral to secondary care, so that treatment with potentially disease modifying agents can be started early—before irreversible joint damage has occurred. For patients with non-inflammatory conditions, such as osteoarthritis and regional or widespread musculoskeletal pain, optimal management depends on the development of efficient triage systems that identify patients with "red flags" who will benefit from referral to secondary care for further investigation and management. Healthcare professionals in primary care should give first line management with the strategies outlined for the rest of patients.

1 Carr A, Gordon T, eds. Defining the extended clinical role for allied health professionals in rheumatology. ARC conference proceedings no 12. Chesterfield: Arthritis Research Campaign, 2001
2 White C, Cooper RG. Prescribing and monitoring of disease-modifying anti-rheumatic drugs (DMARDs) for inflammatory arthritis. *Rheumatic Disease: In Practice*, 2002;8
3 Doherty M, Dougados M, eds. Osteoarthritis: Current Treatment Strategies. *Bailliére's Best Pract Res Clin Rheumatol* 2001;15:517-24
4 Main CJ, Williams A. ABC of psychological medicine: musculoskeletal pain. *BMJ* 2002;325;534-7
5 Hay EM, Dziedic K, Sim J. Treatment options for musculoskeletal pain: what is the evidence? *Bailliére's Clin Rheumatol* 1999;13:243-59

Evidence-based summary

- Early aggressive treatment of rheumatoid arthritis with disease modifying drugs improves clinical outcome and slows radiological progression
- Psychosocial factors are the main predictors of chronic pain disability
- Local steroid injections provide effective short-term relief for soft tissue problems but do not improve long-term outcome

---

Further reading

- O'Dell JR. Combinations of conventional disease modifying antirheumatic drugs. *Rheum Dis Clin North Am* 2001;27:415-26
- Linton SJ. A review of psychological factors in back and neck pain. *Spine* 2000;25:1148-56
- Smidt N, Assendelft WJJ, Windt van der DAWM, Hay EM, Buchbinder R, Bouter L. Corticosteroid injections for lateral epicondylitis: a systematic review. *Pain* 2002;96:23-40

2 Pain in the wrist and hand

Michael A Shipley

Trauma is the most common cause of pain in the wrist and hand. A careful history and examination is essential for accurate diagnosis. "Boggy" swelling around affected joints or tendon sheaths is caused by synovitis. Flexor tendons may be thickened or nodular. Skin changes occur in scleroderma and diabetes, as may vasculitis. X ray examinations help exclude fracture after trauma and are useful in the differential diagnosis of established inflammatory arthritis, but they are usually normal in early arthritis. The patient's work and hobbies may be relevant. Hand or wrist pain is often the cause of great anxiety.

Functional anatomy

The distal radius and triangular cartilage articulate with the proximal carpal bones (scaphoid, lunate, and triquetral) to form the wrist joint, the cavity of which is contiguous with the intercarpal joints. The wrist joints allow dorsal and palmar flexion, and ulnar and radial deviation. Pronation and supination occur at the distal radioulnar and proximal radiohumeral joints. The muscles of the forearm work together to perform movements and in opposition to stabilise the joints. The flexor retinaculum and an arch of carpal bones provide the boundary for the carpal tunnel, which contains the superficial and deep finger flexor tendons and the median nerve. A common synovial tendon sheath extends from a position just proximal to the wrist to the middle of the palm. The flexor pollicis longus and flexor carpi ulnaris have individual sheaths. The ulnar nerve lies under the transverse carpal ligament in Guyon's canal. The finger extensor tendons share a synovial sheath (fourth compartment) under the extensor retinaculum. Extensor pollicis longus and abductor pollicis brevis share the first compartment and run across the radial styloid.

The metacarpal bones articulate with the proximal carpal bones. The thumb moves at the first carpometacarpal and trapezo-scaphoid joints, which are prone to osteoarthritis. The flexor pollicis brevis is attached to the base of the proximal phalanx of the thumb by a tendon that contains a sesamoid bone. The deep and superficial finger flexor tendons have individual synovial sheaths from the middle of the palm to the finger. Flexor pollicis longus has its own sheath, normally extending to the thumb. During flexion, five fibrous bands or pulleys hold the flexor sheaths down. Longitudinal and transverse components of the palmar aponeurosis lie between the tendon sheaths and the palmar skin.

The second to fifth metacarpophalangeal joints flex to about 90°. Active extension is rarely more than 30°. Passive extension varies from 60° to more than 100° in people with hypermobility. The proximal and distal interphalangeal joints are hinge joints. The lumbricals and interossei produce complex movements that involve extension of the interphalangeal joints and flexion at the metacarpophalangeal joints and are essential to fine hand functions, such as writing.

Local corticosteroid injection technique
An injection of local anaesthetic (or topical anaesthetic) is followed by 0·2-1 ml of a suitable steroid preparation, such as

Causes of pain in the wrist and hand

At all ages
- Trauma
- Flexor tenosynovitis
    Carpal tunnel syndrome
- Flexor tendonosis
    Trigger finger or thumb
- De Quervain's tenosynovitis
- Extensor tenosynovitis
- Ganglion
- Cubital tunnel syndrome
- Inflammatory arthritis
- Raynaud's syndrome
- Writer's cramp
- Chronic upper limb pain
- Reflex sympathetic dystrophy
- Scaphoid fracture
- Osteonecrosis

In older patients
- Nodal osteoarthritis
    Distal interphalangeal joints
    First carpometacarpal joints
    Proximal interphalangeal joints
- Scaphoid fracture
- Pseudogout
- Gout
    Acute
    Chronic tophaceous
- Dupuytren's contracture
- Diabetic stiff hand

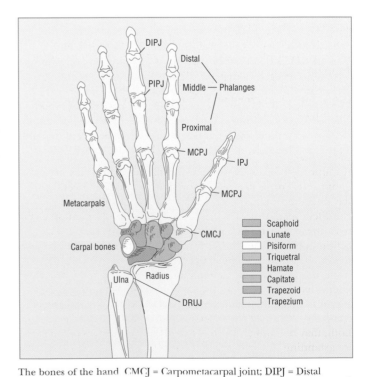

The bones of the hand. CMCJ = Carpometacarpal joint; DIPJ = Distal interphalangeal joint; DRUJ = Distal radio-ulnar joint; IPJ = Interphalangeal joint; MCPJ = Metacarpophalangeal joint; PIPJ = Proximal interphalangeal joint

hydrocortisone acetate 25 mg/ml or depot methylprednisolone 40 mg/ml. Methylprednisolone is about five times as powerful as hydrocortisone on a mg per mg basis. It is best first to introduce the needle with local anaesthetic and then to inject the steroid under low pressure. Patients should be warned that the pain might increase for a day or two after injection. Superficial injections or, very rarely, leakage of the corticosteroid along the needle track, cause local skin depigmentation and atrophy of subcutaneous fat; this is more likely with depot injections of steroid.

Tendon problems

Flexor tenosynovitis
Unaccustomed or repetitive use of the finger and inflammatory arthritis cause inflammation of the synovial sheath of the finger flexor tendons, which leads to volar swelling and tenderness just proximal and distal to the wrist. The flexor tendon sheaths in the palm or finger also may be affected. The hand feels stiff, painful, and swollen, particularly in the morning. Rest helps. A local corticosteroid injection into the tendon sheath is sometimes needed.

Carpal tunnel syndrome
Carpal tunnel syndrome is a peripheral nerve entrapment syndrome often caused by flexor tenosynovitis; it also can occur in the third trimester of pregnancy. Repetitive use of the hand increases the risk of developing carpal tunnel syndrome. Its status as a work injury is controversial.[1] Rarely, a ganglion, amyloidosis, or myxoedema causes carpal tunnel syndrome. Pain, tingling, and numbness in a median nerve distribution (thumb, index, middle, and radial side of ring fingers)—typically are present on waking or can wake the patient. The fingers feel swollen and intense aching is felt in the forearm. The symptoms may appear when the patient holds a newspaper. Permanent numbness and wasting of the thenar eminence (flexor pollicis and opponens pollicis) cause clumsiness. The patient's history often indicates the diagnosis.[2]

Tests and investigations
Tinel's sign (tapping the median nerve in the carpal tunnel) or Phalen's test (holding the wrist in forced dorsiflexion) provoke symptoms. Weakness of abduction of the thumb distal phalanx with the thumb adducted towards the fifth digit is typical. The carpal tunnel and median nerve are seen on ultrasonic images (as well as magnetic resonance images, although these are rarely needed).

Management
A splint worn on the wrist at night relieves or reduces the symptoms. This is diagnostic and may be curative. Recurrent daytime symptoms, unrelieved by splints, warrant nerve conduction studies. Slowing of median nerve conduction at the wrist suggests demyelination due to local compression. The action potential is reduced or absent due to nerve fibre loss if the lesion is severe or prolonged. Needle electromyography is unpleasant but detects denervation. Significant nerve damage needs decompression surgery as a day case or endoscopic surgery.[3] Pins and needles often worsen briefly postoperatively while the nerve recovers. Recovery of sensation or strength, or both, may be limited or non-existent if the lesion is severe and longstanding. A corticosteroid injection into the carpal tunnel often helps rapidly, although recurrence is common, so surgery is usually the first option, except in pregnant women.

The needle is inserted at the distal wrist skin crease, just to the ulnar side of the palmaris longus tendon, or about 0.5 cm

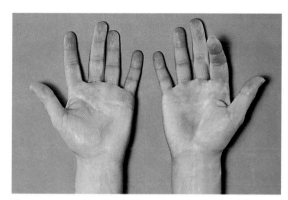

Flexor tenosynovitis

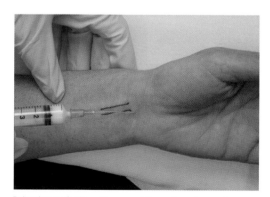

Injection technique for carpal tunnel syndrome

to the ulnar side of flexor carpi radialis at an angle of 45°
towards the middle finger. The local anaesthetic is injected
superficially. If a small test injection of corticosteroid causes
finger pain, the needle is in the nerve and needs to be
repositioned. An injection of 1 ml of corticosteroid
(hydrocortisone acetate 25 mg) often precipitates the
symptoms, but it is effective and non-toxic.[4,5]

Finger flexor tendonosis and trigger finger

Gripping and hard manual work cause palpable thickening and
nodularity of the finger flexor tendon; tendon sheath synovitis
may also be present. The affected fingers are stiff in the
morning, when the paitent also has pain in the palm and along
the dorsum of the finger(s). The pain is reproduced by passive
extension of the finger. This is common in rheumatoid arthritis
and in dactylitis caused by seronegative arthritis. Nodular flexor
tenosynovitis is more common and less responsive to treatment
in patients with diabetes than other patients.[6] A nodule that
catches at the pulley that overlies the metacarpophalangeal joint
in the palm causes trigger finger—the patient wakens with the
finger flexed and has to force it straight with a painful or
painless click. Triggering also occurs after gripping. The nodule
and the "catch" in movement are felt in the palm. A low
pressure corticosteroid injection (hydrocortisone acetate
12.5 mg) alongside the tendon nodule in the palm helps.[7] If
symptoms are persistent or recurrent, surgical release is needed.

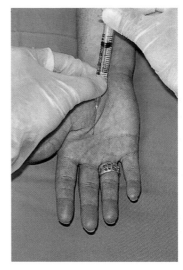

Injection technique for flexor
tenosynovitis and trigger finger

Thumb flexor tenosynovitis and trigger thumb

Overuse and local injury (after opening a tight jar) are the
most common causes. Either the interphalangeal joint cannot
be flexed or it sticks in flexion and snaps straight. The
sesamoid bone in flexor pollicis brevis tendon is tender on the
volar surface of the thumb's metacarpophalangeal joint.
Corticosteroid injection next to the sesamoid bone at the site of
maximal tenderness helps.

De Quervain's tenosynovitis

De Quervain's stenosing tenosynovitis affects the tendon sheath
of abductor pollicis longus and extensor pollicis brevis at the
radial styloid. Pain occurs at or just proximal or distal to the
styloid, in contrast with first carpometacarpal osteoarthritis,
which causes pain at the base of the thumb. Tenderness,
swelling, and pushing the thumb into the palm—Finkelstein's
test—increase the pain. Crepitus or a tendon nodule may cause
triggering.

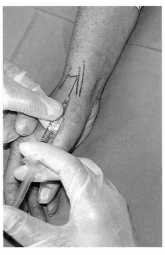

Injection technique for de Quervain's
tenosynovitis

Management
Rest is essential, with avoidance of thumb extension and
pinching, but immobilisation splints are inconvenient.
Therapeutic ultrasound or local anti-inflammatory gels help;
injection of hydrocortisone acetate 25 mg alongside the tendon
under low pressure at the point of maximum tenderness
rapidly relieves pain. A second injection may be needed.
Surgery is rarely necessary unless stenosis or nodule formation
develops.

Extensor tenosynovitis

Inflammation of the common extensor (fourth) compartment
causes well defined swelling that extends from the back of the
hand to just proximal to the wrist. The extensor retinaculum
causes a typical "hourglass" shape proximal and distal to the
wrist. This contrasts with wrist synovitis, which causes diffuse
swelling distal to the radius and ulna. Rest helps extensor
tenosynovitis but often a corticosteroid injection into the tendon
sheath is needed. Workplace reviews and wrist supports for those
who use a keyboard and mouse help prevent recurrences.

> **Repetitive wrist and finger movements,
> especially with the wrist in dorsiflexion, are
> the cause and this is one of the several
> causes of forearm and wrist pain seen in
> keyboard workers. It also is common in
> rheumatoid arthritis**

Osteoarthritis

Nodal osteoarthritis

Nodal osteoarthritis most commonly involves the distal interphalangeal joints and is familial. The joint swells and becomes inflamed and painful, but the pain subsides over a few weeks or months and leaves bony swellings (Heberden's nodes). Most patients manage with local anti-inflammatory gels or no treatment once they know the prognosis is good. The appearance sometimes causes distress. Occasionally, the joint becomes unstable. Surgical fusion of the index distal interphalangeal joints or thumb interphalangeal joint in slight flexion improves pinch gripping. Involvement of the proximal interphalangeal joints (Bouchard's node) is less common. It may be mistaken for early rheumatoid arthritis. Stiffness of the proximal joints impairs hand function significantly.

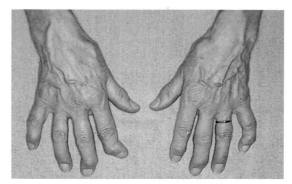

Nodal osteoarthritis (Heberden's nodes) and first carpometacarpal osteoarthritis

First carpometacarpal osteoarthritis

Pain at the base of the thumb in the early phase of first carpometacarpal osteoarthritis is disabling, but with time the joint stiffens and adducts, and pain and disability decrease. The hand becomes "squared." Management is usually conservative, but a corticosteroid injection helps severe pain. Surgical replacement is rarely warranted, although the outcome is good.

Dupuytren's contracture

This relatively common and painless condition is associated with palpable fibrosis of the palmar aponeurosis, usually in the palm but occasionally at the base of a digit. It is more common in white people, men, heavy drinkers, smokers, and patients with diabetes mellitus. The cause is unknown, but repeated trauma may be important. Fibroblast proliferation starts in the superficial fascia and invades the dermis. An early sign is skin pitting or puckering. The contraction eventually causes flexion of the digit(s), most often the ring finger, but disability is often minimal. Disabling and progressive flexion is more common in the familial form. Nodular fibromatosis also affects the sole of the foot, the knuckle pads (Garrod's pads), and the penis (Peyronie's disease), and the two conditions may coexist. Specialist hand clinics use magnetic resonance imaging to assess the lesion. The role of local corticosteroid injections and radiotherapy in early disease is unclear.[8,9] Surgical excision is helpful but recurrence is common. No controlled studies exist.

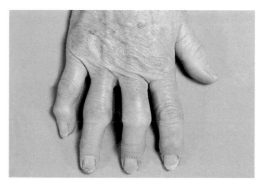

Nodal osteoarthritis with Bouchard's nodes

Cubital tunnel syndrome

Ulnar nerve compression at the elbow can be caused by direct pressure from leaning on the elbow, stretching the nerve with the elbow in prolonged flexion at night, or holding a telephone. It causes pins and needles in the ulnar side of the hand. Prolonged entrapment causes hypothenar wasting and weakness of the hand's intrinsic muscles. The nerve is tender and sensitive at the elbow, where Tinel's sign is positive. Nerve conduction studies are normal in around 50% of cases. Avoidance of direct pressure and prolonged elbow flexion help. Surgical anterior transposition of the nerve is occasionally needed. In some cases the ulnar nerve is compressed in Guyon's canal at the wrist.

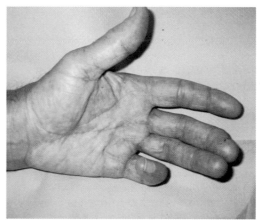

Dupuytren's contracture

Systemic disorders causing hand pain

Inflammatory arthritis

In rheumatoid arthritis the metacarpophalangeal joints, proximal interphalangeal joints, and wrists are affected. Psoriatic and other forms of seronegative arthritis are less common, are more likely to be asymmetrical, and may

Rheumatoid arthritis often affects the hands early in the disease, usually symmetrically, and involves the feet and other joints

be associated with marked skin and tendon changes that produce a "sausage" finger. The distal interphalangeal joints and adjacent nails may also be affected in psoriasis. Morning pain and stiffness are typical. Intra-articular steroids are often useful adjuncts to systemic medication.

Acute pseudogout and chondrocalcinosis

Sudden wrist inflammation in an older patient may be due to calcium pyrophosphate arthritis (pseudogout). Marked swelling and inflammation are found—the joint feels hot, and infection may need to be excluded. Chondrocalcinosis, although often asymptomatic, is usually seen in the triangular ligament of the wrist on x ray radiography. The joint aspirate is turbid and contains weakly positively birefringent crystals under polarised light. Steroid injection or a short course of a non-steroidal anti-inflammatory drug usually helps; regular use of non-steroidal anti-inflammatory drugs can be used to manage frequent attacks.

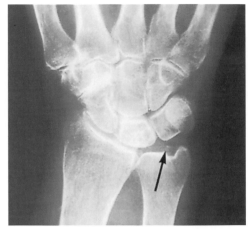

Chondrocalcinosis in wrist

Diabetic stiff hand (cheiroarthropathy—limited joint mobility syndrome)

Stiff hands are seen in 5-10% of patients with type I diabetes. This is more common in those with poor diabetic control and is associated with limited shoulder mobility, diabetic nephropathy, and retinopathy. Patients develop waxy and tight skin. Limited joint mobility in diabetes is multifactorial, however, and may also be due to flexor tenosynovitis, Dupuytren's contracture, or nodal osteoarthritis.[10] Good diabetic control is essential. Injection of symptomatic flexor tenosynovitis helps. No specific treatment exists for the skin changes.

Raynaud's phenomenon

This disorder, which results from severe vasospasm in response to a temperature change, causes marked and typically sharply demarcated pallor of one or more digits. As circulation recovers, the digit becomes blue (cyanotic) and then bright red because of rebound hyperaemia—the triphasic response. In young women the condition is often a harmless nuisance, requiring warm gloves and sometimes vasodilators. Its onset in older people, especially, is more often pathological. It may also be part of a systemic autoimmune disorder (rheumatoid arthritis, systemic lupus erythematosus, or systemic sclerosis), and it occasionally leads to necrosis. It requires specialist referral. Vibration white finger is a compensatable industrial disease in people who use vibrating tools.

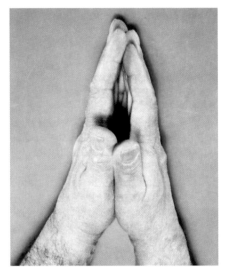

Positive prayer sign—diabetic stiff hands (also nodal osteoarthritis and flexor tenosynovitis)

Other disorders

Ganglion

A ganglion is a cystic swelling in continuity with a joint or tendon sheath through a fault in the capsule. It is filled with clear, viscous fluid rich in hyaluronan. Ganglia are common on the dorsal wrist, are often painless and resolve spontaneously. Wrist splints relieve the pain. Injection is rarely effective, and surgical excision is best if the ganglion is persistent and painful.

Chronic (work-related) upper limb pain

The main symptom is pain. A local cause (carpal tunnel syndrome, flexor or extensor tenosynovitis, or tennis elbow) may be the initial trigger. The patient develops widespread pain that is often disproportionate to the findings but causes great distress. A prior change in work pattern may exist, and often disharmony is found at the workplace. The cause is unclear, but neurophysiological and psychosocial factors are probably involved. The phenomenon of central "wind up" of pain seen

> **Infective arthritis is a medical emergency and should be referred to a specialist unit or emergency department**

Characteristics of chronic upper limb pain syndrome

- Often starts as carpal tunnel syndrome, flexor tenosynovitis, or tennis elbow
- Spreads to affect the upper arm more diffusely
- Physical signs may be minimal
- Often associated with:
    Use of keyboards
    Sudden changes in work practices
    Disharmony at work
    Anxiety and sleeplessness
- Neurophysiological and psychosocial mechanisms involved
- Best dealt with non-judgmentally

---

in many chronic pain syndromes probably plays a role. It is easy for the doctor to find the problem exasperating and difficult to understand, but it is best managed non-judgmentally. Early reductions in work activities and pain control measures are important, but it is best not to ask the person to take too much time off. Advice to the employer to review work practices reduces the risk of litigation. Referral to a specialist pain clinic should be considered.

Osteonecrosis (rare)

Kienboeck disease is the late result of a dorsiflexion injury often seen in manual labourers. Fragmentation and collapse of the lunate causes shortening of the carpus and secondary osteoarthritis. Osteonecrosis takes up to 18 months to appear on x ray radiography.

Scaphoid bone fracture

Pain in the anatomical snuffbox after a fall onto an outstretched hand requires an immediate x ray examination although a fracture is not always visible. Any severe wrist injury should be managed as a potential scaphoid fracture with a plaster, and a further x ray radiograph should be taken three weeks later. Unrecognised scaphoid fracture leads to pain associated with failed union, osteonecrosis, and secondary osteoarthritis.

Writer's cramp

Writer's cramp is the most common type of focal dystonia and occurs during complex hand activities—writing or playing a musical instrument. Clumsiness and painful tightness in the hand and forearm occur during writing or playing, and abnormal tension and strange posturing develop. Dystonias are often inappropriately described as "psychological." Local botulinum toxin injection produces temporary relief. Retraining and learning new techniques help some patients, but the outlook is poor and may lead to the end of musical careers.

1 Yagev Y, Carel RS, Yagev R. Assessment of work-related risk factors for carpal tunnel syndrome. *Isr Med Assoc J* 2001;3:569-71
2 Pal B, O'Gradaigh D, Merry P. Diagnosis of carpal tunnel syndrome. *Rheumatology* 2001;40:595-7
3 Trumble TE, Gilbert M, McCallister WV. Endoscopic versus open surgical treatment of carpal tunnel syndrome. *Neurosurg Clin N Am* 2001;12:255-66
4 Wong SM, Hui ACF, O'Gradaigh D, Merry P. Corticosteroid injection for the treatment of carpal tunnel syndrome. *Ann Rheum Dis* 2001;60:897
5 O'Gradaigh D, Merry P. Corticosteroid injection for the treatment of carpal tunnel syndrome. *Ann Rheum Dis* 2000;59:918-19
6 Stahl S, Kanter Y, Karnelli E. Outcome of trigger finger treatment in diabetes. *J Rheumatol* 1997;24:931-6
7 Rankin ME, Rankin EA. Injection therapy for management of stenosing tenosynovitis (de Quervain's disease) of the wrist. *J Natl Med Assoc* 1998;90:474-6
8 Ketchum LD, Donahue TK. The injection of nodules of Dupuytren's disease with triamcinolone acetonide. *J Hand Surg (Am)* 2000;25:1157-62
9 Seegenschmiedt MH, Olschewski T, Guntrum F. Radiotherapy optimization in early-stage Dupuytren's contracture; results of a randomized study. *Int J Radiat Oncol Biol Phys* 2001;49:785-98
10 Griggs SM, Weiss AP, Lane LB, Schwenker C, Akelman E, Sachar K. Treatment of trigger finger in patients with diabetes mellitus. *J Hand Surg (Am)* 1995;20:787-9

The picture of the bones of the hand is adapted from teaching material on the website www.pncl.co.uk/~belcher/home.htm

3 Pain in the neck, shoulder, and upper arm

Cathy Speed

The neck and shoulder are two of the most common sources of musculoskeletal pain. Overall, 71% of the general population experience neck pain that persists for more than three months at some stage in their lives, with a point prevalence of 9.5% of men and 13.5% of women. Risk factors include manual jobs, heavy workloads, increasing age, and depression. Shoulder pain has a point prevalence of up to 21% in community dwelling adults; the incidence and functional impact increase with age.

The neck moves almost constantly during waking hours through flexion, extension, and rotation at the intervertebral and facet joints of the seven cervical vertebrae, through the actions of the surrounding muscles. Vital neurovascular structures are protected by the vertebrae.

The shoulder is a series of articulations including the scapulothoracic articulation, where the scapula slides on the rib cage. Soft tissue structures—capsules, ligaments, muscles, tendons, bursae, and neurovascular elements—complete the framework and allow remarkable mobility to be achieved, which is important to function. The glenohumeral joint is extremely mobile and relies on the rotator cuff for stability. Instability, caused by laxity (congenital or acquired) or lack of muscular control because of pain, is a common feature of shoulder complaints.

The elbow is a compound synovial joint composed of a complex of two closely related articulations between the humerus and both the ulna and radius. It is supported by the ligaments and muscles.

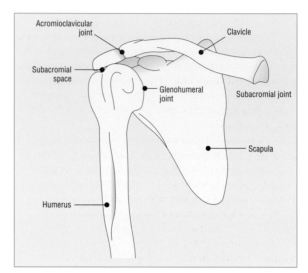

The shoulder "complex" of joints. This includes the scapulothoracic articulation, where the scapula slides on the rib cage

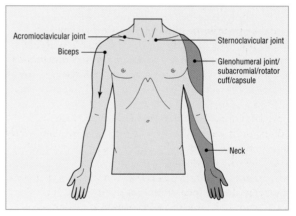

Sites and radiation of pain in the shoulder, arm, and neck

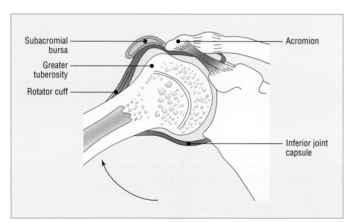

Subacromial impingement of the rotator cuff can occur with abduction of the arm

Clinical evaluation

As neck and arm pain have a wide differential diagnosis, a detailed history is vital to make a correct diagnosis and, where possible, determine the cause. Details of the patient's expectations, hand dominance, occupation, hobbies, past medical history, functional disability, and previous treatments should be noted.

The cardinal symptom is usually pain, and a carefully taken history of the pain will determine the mode of onset, nature, site, radiation, temporal characteristics, exacerbating and relieving features, and associated symptoms. Nocturnal pain is not uncommon in substantial soft tissue complaints, but it

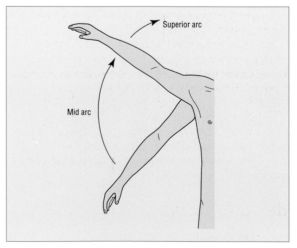

Mid or superior painful arcs of abduction represent subacromial impingement or acromioclavicular pathology, respectively

should raise suspicion of nerve root pain, bony pathology, or underlying malignancy. Radiation of pain from the upper arm or elbow suggests referred pain from the neck or peripheral neurological lesions. Neurological symptoms should be sought and their distribution ascertained. Weakness can also arise because of pain or a rotator cuff tear.

Other notable symptoms include stiffness, clicking, clunking, crunching, or locking. Joint swelling around the shoulder or elbow can occur in relation to arthropathy, infection, or trauma. Systemic symptoms should be addressed specifically, because of the possibility of infection, malignancy, or other systemic disease. The duration and progression of symptoms indicate the severity of the condition and are used to plan its management.

A structured examination aims to define the source of the pain and the degree of functional deficit and coexisting pathologies. It should include careful inspection, palpation, movement, special tests, neurological assessment, and further examination, as appropriate.

Plain radiographs are useful in patients with neck or shoulder pain, when bony pathology or inflammatory arthritis is suspected, but radiographic abnormalities in the neck and shoulder often do not correlate well with clinical features.

X ray examinations of the shoulder (anteroposterior and axial views) may also show subacromial osteophytes or calcification in the cuff. Ultrasound imaging and magnetic resonance imaging are valuable in the assessment of soft tissue structures of the shoulder and arm. Magnetic resonance imaging is highly sensitive in the detection of disc and cord abnormalities, whereas computed tomography is better for evaluation of bone.

Disorders of the cervical spine

Pain in the neck can arise because of disorders within the components of the spine, may be referred from elsewhere, or, most commonly, may be because of poorly defined mechanical influences upon the neck ("mechanical" or "non-specific" neck pain). This is often suggested by the history and the presence or absence of localising signs.

Neck pain is common in inflammatory arthritis and atlantoaxial and subaxial subluxation are concerns, particularly in rheumatoid arthritis. Immobility due to osteophytic linking of vertebrae is seen in ankylosing spondylitis.

Radicular pain usually arises because of a prolapsed cervical disc, but it may be due to local infection or tumour. Typical neurological features are evident and magnetic resonance imaging confirms the diagnosis. Although rehabilitation may be successful, surgery may be necessary.

Whiplash as a result of rapid acceleration or deceleration can be characterised by quite localised or diffuse neck and arm pain with muscle spasm.

Myofascial pain is suggested by regional pain that is reproduced by palpation of trigger points ("knots" within muscle). Management includes physiotherapy, dry needling of the trigger point, and use of a tricyclic agent.

Mechanical or non-specific neck pain may be responsive to heat packs, simple analgesics, non-steroidal anti-inflammatory drugs, taping, exercise therapy and stretching, and correction of postural deficiencies and other provocative factors. Symptoms may also respond to a tricyclic antidepressant taken at night, acupuncture, or local facet blocks.

Shoulder disorders

Generalised shoulder pain
Most shoulder complaints are due to extra-articular disorders, with rotator cuff lesions (tendinosis and tears) the most

Features of cervical nerve root lesions

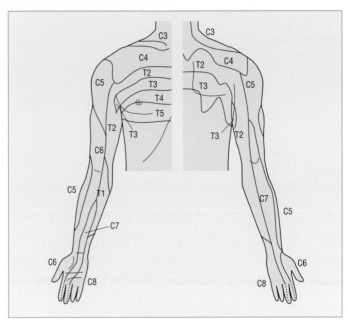

Arm dermatomes

Nerve root	Weakness	Reflex change
C5	Shoulder abduction	Biceps
C6	Wrist extension, supination, elbow flexion	Radial
C7	Elbow extension, wrist flexion	Triceps
C8	Finger flexors	NA
T1	Finger abductors	NA

Note NA = not applicable

Differential diagnosis of neck pain

Structural
- Mechanical or non-specific
- Facet joint arthritis or dysfunction
- Prolapsed intervertebral disc

Neoplasm
- Primary or secondary

Inflammatory
- Rheumatoid arthritis
- Spondyloarthropathies

Infection
- Discitis
- Osteomyelitis
- Paraspinal abcess

Muscular
- Polymyalgia rheumatica
- Polymyositis

Metabolic
- Paget's disease

Myofascial
- Myofascial syndromes, fibromyalgia

common complaint. The most common cause is impingement upon the cuff by subacromial osteophytes or instability, the latter being particularly common in younger or active patients. Longstanding tears can result in glenohumeral arthritis (cuff arthropathy).

The patient typically complains of global shoulder pain that is worse with overhead activities and at night, particularly when they lie on the affected side. Examination may reveal wasting of the spinati, evidence of impingement, and pain on resisted testing of the cuff, with weakness if a substantial tear is present. Management aims to control pain to allow rehabilitation to proceed, including re-education and strengthening of shoulder movements. Pain control may be achieved through modification of activities, heat or ice packs, simple analgesics, non-steroidal anti-inflammatory drugs, a tricyclic agent, or a subacromial corticosteroid injection—although the latter is best avoided in younger patients. In appropriate resistant cases, surgery to remove subacromial osteophytes is often effective.

Calcifying tendinitis—A distinct, transient form of rotator cuff tendinopathy that usually affects women aged 30-50 years and is associated with the formation and resorption of calcific deposits within the cuff. A dull ache in the shoulder is followed by acute and constant pain, occasionally with a fever. The patient may appear unwell and guard the affected arm in internal rotation, with shoulder movements globally restricted by pain. In the more chronic stages, pain and catching are reported, and signs of impingement may be noted. Investigations exclude other causes of shoulder pain with systemic symptoms. The erythrocyte sedimentation rate and white cell count may be raised, and typical calcification, which differs from that associated with articular disease, may be noted on x ray radiography.

Treatment involves pain control with rest and support of the affected arm, regular ice packs, or analgesics or non-steroidal anti-inflammatory drugs, or both. Treatment is followed by gentle mobilisation, and then by progressive stretching and strengthening exercises. Conventional ultrasound, shock wave therapy, subacromial injection of corticosteroid, or needling of the most symptomatic areas under fluoroscopic control can all be effective. Surgical removal of deposits is reserved for those with protracted symptoms.

Frozen shoulder—Also called adhesive capsulitis, this affects 2-3% of the population, but it is rare before the age of 40 years. The incidence may be as high as 35% in patients with diabetes, in whom it is more severe. An acute inflammatory process results in synovitis, fibroplasias, and then capsular contracture. The initial painful phase involves shoulder pain, which is often worse at night. Restriction progresses in the adhesive and resolution phases, when the pain eases. Gradual improvement in mobility is usually seen, but recovery commonly takes 12-42 months. Examination reveals passive and active restriction of shoulder movements, often mild wasting of the spinati and deltoid, and signs of impingement. Blood tests are normal. X ray examination excludes glenohumeral arthritis.

Treatment aims to control pain and promote function through gradual mobilisation and strengthening exercises. Analgesics, a tricyclic agent, non-steroidal anti-inflammatory drugs, corticosteroids (articular injection or two weeks of oral prednisolone 7.5-15 mg), and suprascapular nerve blockade are common approaches. Distension of the joint or manipulation under anaesthesia is considered in intractable cases.

Glenohumeral joint arthritides—These include osteoarthritis, inflammatory and crystal arthritides, and sepsis. All of these

Differential diagnosis of general shoulder pain

Site	Lesions
Rotator cuff	• Tendinosis, impingement
	• Calcifying tendinitis
	• Tear
	• Global rupture
Tendon of long head of biceps	• Tendinosis, impingement
	• Calcifying tendinitis
	• Tear or rupture
Capsule	• Frozen shoulder
Joint complex and surrounding musculature	• Glenohumeral instabilities, labral lesions
Bursae	• Subacromial, subdeltoid, bursitis
Nerves	• Lesions of axillary, suprascapular, long thoracic, radial, musculocutaneous nerves, brachial plexus, referred pain
Muscle	• Myofascial pain syndromes
Joint	• Glenohumeral arthritides
Others	• Local destructive lesions

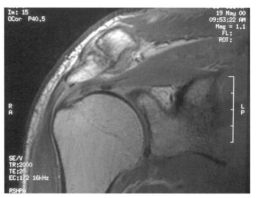

MRI scan of shoulder showing acromioclavular osteophytes and underlying rotator cuff tendinitis

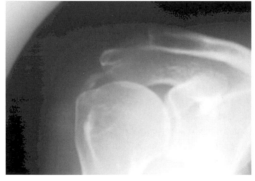

A plain x ray showing calcifying tendinitis

Lesions associated with frozen shoulder

Primary
• Idiopathic

Secondary
• Shoulder trauma (including surgery)
• Neurological lesions (for example hemiplegia)
• Diabetes mellitus (types 1 and 2)
• Hypoactive or hyperactive thyroid disease
• Cardiac disease or surgery
• Pulmonary disorders

have typical investigative findings and follow the management protocols as used at other sites.

Glenoid labrum (cartilage) injuries—These can cause persistent shoulder pain and instability, and they usually occur after an episode of trauma or dislocation or with overuse. Diagnosis can be difficult, requiring magnetic resonance arthrography or arthroscopy. Management involves pain control and rehabilitation, which is followed by surgery if necessary.

Neurological causes—Shoulder pain may result from neurological causes including nerve root entrapment at the neck, brachial plexus lesions, or peripheral nerve lesions, including the axillary, long thoracic, suprascapular, radial, or musculocutaneous nerves.

Brachial neuritis—This can affect one or more components of the brachial plexus. Often idiopathic, some cases occur after a viral infection (with herpes zoster or Epstein-Barr viruses), immunisations, or mechanical trauma or in relation to autoimmune disease. A sudden onset of diffuse pain in the shoulder, upper arm, and occasionally forearm, is accompanied by weakness, wasting, scapular winging, and variable sensory loss of the affected neuromuscular structures. Electromyographic studies are confirmatory. Non-steroidal anti-inflammatory drugs are usually ineffective, but a tricyclic agent, carbemazapine, or both, is helpful. Rehabilitation is started early to prevent stiffness and improve function.

Thoracic outlet syndrome—This results from compression of the neurovascular structures of the thoracic outlet, brachial plexus, and subclavian artery. Local masses and anatomical variations may be involved—such as a high first or cervical rib or fibrous bands. Symptoms of thoracic outlet syndrome depend on the structures compressed, but they usually are exacerbated by heavy manual work. Neurogenic symptoms usually predominate, including aching in the arm, paraesthesiae, and weakness. Vascular symptoms are usually intermittent cyanosis; trophic skin changes can occur. Although imaging (computed tomography, magnetic resonance imaging, and vascular studies) is often pursued, a causative structure is rarely identified and management is symptomatic.

Localised shoulder pain

Acromioclavicular joint disorders

Acromioclavicular joint disorders consist of sprains due to trauma and arthritides. Sprains are managed with taping, analgesia, and in severe cases, surgery. Osteoarthritis of the acromioclavicular joint is extremely common and is managed symptomatically with analgesics. Local corticosteroid injections can provide relief. Surgery can be effective in resistant cases.

The sternoclavicular joint can be the presenting site of an inflammatory arthritis, but it is frequently overlooked. Osteoarthritis and sepsis can also occur. Instability, with pain or clunking, can occur after trauma, or spontaneously in younger patients. Treatment of the latter should be symptomatic.

Elbow and forearm pain

Lateral epicondylitis

This is in fact a degenerative tendinopathy of the common extensor–supinator tendon, which is related to repetitive flexion–extension or pronation–supination of the forearm. It is characterised by lateral peri-epicondylar pain and tenderness that are exacerbated by gripping and stressing the tendon. The differential diagnosis of lateral elbow pain is wide and there is a tendency to overdiagnose lateral epicondylitis.

Treatment in the acute stage involves relative rest, use of a compression strap or counterforce brace, ice, analgesics, and (preferably topical) non-steroidal anti-inflammatory drugs. In non-acute cases, transverse friction massage helps to break down

---

Differential diagnosis of scapulothoracic pain

- Local muscle injury
- Myofascial pain syndrome
- Subscapular bursitis
- Snapping scapula
- Suprascapular nerve palsy
- Referred pain from cervical or thoracic spine
- Bony injury—for example, fracture or metastatic deposit in scapula

---

Differential diagnosis of elbow pain

Lateral elbow pain

Tendon	• Lateral epicondylitis
Ligament	• Instability
Bursa	• Radiocapitellar bursitis
Nerve	• C6 root pathology, radial nerve lesions
Bone	• Epicondylar apophysitis (adolescents)
Vascular	• Forearm compartment syndrome

Medial elbow pain

Tendon	• Medial epicondylitis
Ligament	• Ulnar collateral ligament sprain or instability
Nerve	• Cervical radiculopathy
	• Ulnar neuropathy
Bone	• Medial apophysitis

Posterior elbow pain

Tendon	• Triceps tendinopathy, avulsion
Bursa	• Olecranon bursitis
Nerve	• Cervical radiculopathy
Joint	• Osteochondrosis
	• Osteochondritis dissecans
	• Osteoarthritis
Bone	• Traction apophysitis

Anterior elbow pain

Tendon	• Distal biceps tendinopathies
Nerve	• C-spine radiculopathy
	• Median nerve, anterior interosseous nerve, and cubital tunnel syndromes
Vascular	• Forearm compartment syndromes

All

Joint	• Osteochondrosis
	• Osteochondritis dissecans or arthritides
Bone	• Fracture or stress fracture

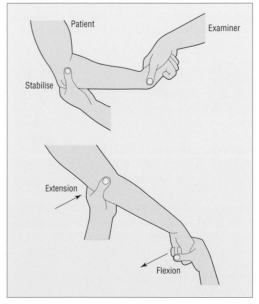

Provocation tests for lateral epicondylitis. Resisted extension of the middle finger also elicits pain

scar tissue. Corticosteroid injections should be limited to those with persistent pain that limits rehabilitation, but subcutaneous atrophy is a risk. Stretching and progressive strengthening of the muscles at the elbow and wrist starts early. The most common cause for persistent symptoms is failure to address the cause—this is particularly an issue in manual workers. Surgery is reserved for patients with recalcitrant, limiting symptoms: a number of techniques have been described.

Medial epicondylitis

This is another degenerative tendinopathy, which affects the common tendinous origin of the flexor–pronator muscle group. It usually occurs because of repetitive flexion or pronation or with valgus stresses. Much less common than lateral epicondylitis, it tends to be overdiagnosed.

Pain and tenderness are found at the medial elbow and proximal flexor musculature of the forearm and are exacerbated by grip and provocation tests. Decreased range of motion at the elbow is due to tightness of the flexor–pronator group. Other causes of medial elbow pain should be considered, particularly if the treatment regimen described for lateral epicondylitis is ineffective. Corticosteroid injections are rarely necessary; caution should be exercised due to the close proximity of the ulnar nerve.

Olecranon bursitis (Student's elbow)

This is caused by acute or repetitive trauma, crystals, or sepsis. Steroid injections precede infections in up to 10% of cases, and the most common causative organism is *Staphylococcus aureus*. Discrete swelling occurs at the posterior elbow, the skin may be inflamed and broken, and a local effusion of the elbow may be present. Systemic upset, leucocytosis, and elevated inflammatory markers occur with sepsis and crystals. When olecranon bursitis is suspected, blood cultures and aspiration for crystals, Gram stain, and culture are essential.

Uncomplicated cases are managed symptomatically. Aspiration without injection can help relieve pain. Steroid injection is reserved for those with inflammatory or crystal arthritis. Broad spectrum antibiotics and possibly open drainage and lavage are used when there is sepsis.

Radiculopathies and peripheral nerve entrapments

These can cause neurological disturbances in the elbow and forearm pain. Nerve conduction studies are helpful in diagnosis. Management depends on the severity and cause, which includes local entrapment and causes of mononeuritis multiplex.

The figures of the glenohumeral joint, the shoulder complex, and the sites of radiation of pain are adapted from the chapter on shoulder disorders. Speed C, Hazleman B, Dalton S. *Fast facts soft tissue rheumatology.* Health Press, 2000. The figure showing provocation tests is adapted from the chapter on elbow disorders in the same book.

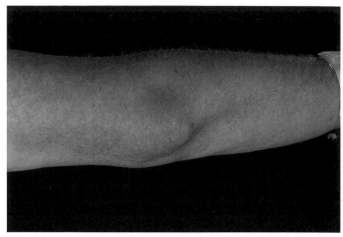

Olecranon bursitis—for example, tophaceous gout at the elbow

Causes of olecranon bursitis

- Trauma (acute or chronic)
- Sepsis
- Metabolic or crystals
- Inflammatory arthritis

- Uraemia
- Calcific deposits
- Idiopathic

Further reading

Examination
- Dalton S. Clinical examination of the painful shoulder. *Baillière's Clin Rheumatol* 1989;3:453-74

Epidemiology
- Bjelle A. Epidemiology of shoulder problems. *Baillière's Clin Rheumatol* 1989;3:437-51

Management
- Binder A. Neck pain. *Clin Evid* 2001;6:884-93
- Speed C, Hazleman B. Shoulder pain. *Clin Evid* 2002;7:1122-39
- Hadler NM. Coping with arm pain in the workplace. *Clin Orthop Rel Res* 1998;351:57-62
- McClune T, Burton AK, Waddell G. Whiplash associated disorders: a review of the literature to guide patient information and advice. *Emerg Med J* 2002;19:499-506

Imaging
- Royal College of Radiologists. *Making the best use of a department of clinical radiology: guidelines for doctors.* London: Royal College of Radiologists, 1999

4 Low back pain

Cathy Speed

Low back pain affects more than 70% of the population in developed countries and poses a major socioeconomic burden, accounting for 13% of sickness absences in the United Kingdom. The annual incidence in adults is up to 45%, with those aged 35-55 years affected most often. In total, 5% of adults present with a new episode each year. Although 90% of episodes of acute low back pain settle within six weeks, up to 7% develop chronic pain.

Causes of low back pain

Low back pain has many causes. It may be due to pathology at one or more sites within the spine itself or it might be a feature of a systemic disease, sepsis, or malignancy. Overall, 1% of people seen with back pain in primary care have a neoplasm, 4% have compression fractures, and 1-3% have a prolapsed disc. Pain may also be referred to the back or from it.

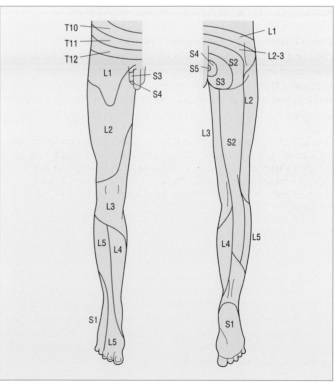

Basic anatomy of the lumbar spine and sacroiliac joints

Causes of low back pain

Structural
- Mechanical or non-specific
- Facet joint arthritis or dysfunction
- Prolapsed intervertebral disc
- Annular tear
- Spondylolysis or spondylolisthesis
- Spinal stenosis

Neoplasm
- Primary or secondary

Referred pain to spine
- From major viscera, retroperitoneal structures, urogenital system, aorta, or hip

Infection
- Discitis
- Osteomyelitis
- Paraspinal abscess

Inflammatory
- Spondyloarthropathies
- Sacroiliitis or sacroiliac dysfunction

Metabolic
- Osteoporotic vertebral collapse
- Paget's disease
- Osteomalacia
- Hyperparathyroidism

Evaluation of patients with pain in the low back

Evaluation of patients with back pain aims first to identify the source of the pain and in particular to identify the few patients who have a serious underlying disorder. Assessment then aims

Features of lumbar and nerve root lesions

Nerve root	Weakness	Reflex change
L2	Hip flexion, adduction	NA
L3	Knee extension	Knee
L4	Knee extension Ankle dorsiflexion	Knee
L5	Foot inversion Great toe dorsiflexion Knee flexion	NA
S1	Ankle plantar flexion Knee flexion	Ankle

Note NA = not applicable

Lumbo-sacral dermatomes

to assess the degree of pain and functional limitation, define the contributing factors where possible, evaluate the patient's expectations, and develop an appropriate management strategy.

A careful history is taken, including: the nature of the onset of the complaint; occupational, sporting, and general medical history; the characteristics of the pain; neurological symptoms; morning stiffness, and systemic features. Typical patterns are suggestive of different pathologies. Suspicion of an underlying complaint should be particularly high when the patient is aged under 20 years or over 55 years at initial onset, when pain is non-mechanical or thoracic, and when systemic symptoms, neurological signs, a structural deformity, or a past history of malignancy, steroids, or HIV are present.

Examination should assess gait, posture, deformities, ease of range, and rhythm of movement, site of pain and tenderness, neurological signs, provoking movements, and contributing factors. Detailed examination of other systems is necessary, because pain may be referred.

Imaging of the lumbar spine

Radiographs of the spine are not usually necessary for patients with back pain, unless an underlying systemic disorder, such as spondyloarthropathy, spondylolysis, infection, or malignancy, is suspected. Computed tomography shows the bony anatomy and also gives the best images of the detail of facet degeneration and spinal stenosis. Magnetic resonance imaging gives insight in particular into soft tissue structures, such as the discs and nerve roots. Isotope bone scanning is indicated in specific situations, such as suspected sacroiliitis or malignancy.

Low back with leg pain

Many spinal complaints can result in pain referred to the leg and in some cases back pain may not be noted. The distribution of leg pain and associated signs offer insight into whether the pain is caused by nerve root entrapment (radiculopathy). True sciatica radiates below the ankle, and if the nerve is stretched, root pain is exacerbated.

The most common cause of true sciatica is intervertebral disc prolapse. Intervertebral discs make up about 25% of the height of the spine. Each disc consists of an outer fibro-cartilagenous annulus fibrosus, which facilitates torsional movements, and an inner nucleus pulposus. The fibres of the annulus are kept under tension by the nucleus pulposus, which is made up of 70-90% water; this allows changes in shape in response to compressive force.

Nerve roots lie in the immediate path of laterally prolapsing intervertebral discs. In the lumbar spine, such prolapses can compress the lower emerging root to produce pain and dysaesthesiae in the associated dermatome and other features typical of a lumbar root syndrome.

Spinal stenosis
Narrowing of the spinal canal is relatively common in the elderly and can have a number of causes, including facet joint arthrosis, ossification of the longitudinal ligament, Paget's disease, and ankylosing spondylitis. Symptoms typically include low back pain, leg pain, and pseudoclaudication. Imaging of the spinal canal with magnetic resonance imaging or computed tomography is needed, and surgery is indicated for those with severe symptoms.

Cauda equina syndrome
Compression of the cauda equina can occur with central disc herniation, epidural masses (for example, abscesses), or

---

Important questions relating to back pain: "PQRST"

Provocative and **P**alliative factors
Quality of pain
Radiation
Severity and **S**ystemic **S**ymptoms
Timing

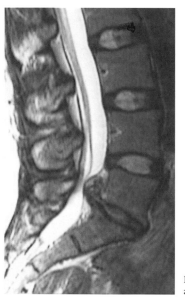

Magnetic resonance image showing a posterolateral disc prolapse

Posture has a profound effect on intradisc pressure; forward flexion is associated with the largest increase in pressure and thus provokes pain

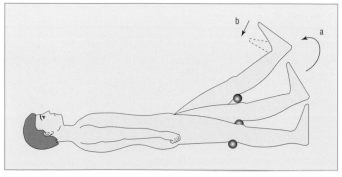

The straight leg raise test is positive if pain in the sciatic distribution is reproduced between 30 and 70° passive flexion of the straight leg. Dorsiflexion of the foot exacerbates the pain

tumours. Low back pain, bilateral sciatica, saddle anaesthesia, loss of sphincter tone, and bladder and bowel incontinence may result. Urgent magnetic resonance imaging is needed to investigate the cause and direct the management.

Facet arthrosis or syndrome

Pain from facet joints is very common, particularly in patients with degenerative disc disease. Local or diffuse back pain may be associated with leg pain but without localising neurological signs. Treatment involves analgesia, modification of activities, and rehabilitation. Local corticosteroid injections are used occasionally.

Non-specific back pain

In 85% of cases, pain in the low back results from the presumed effects of mechanical and postural stresses upon spinal and paraspinal structures ("non-specific" back pain), although the pathophysiology is poorly understood. Relevant mechanical stresses upon the spine include twisting, flexion, extension, rotation, lifting, repetitive work, and static postures, such as sitting at a desk. Muscles, particularly those of the abdomen (the obliques, transversus, and recti) provide dynamic stability and fine control to the spine. This is important when deciding on the appropriate management of non-specific back pain.

Pain can be worse with movement in any plane, may radiate to one or both legs, and is relieved by lying with the hips and knees flexed.

Management

In the absence of serious pathology, the essential features of management are education and encouragement about pain control so that rehabilitation can be started. Pain management can include the short-term use of simple analgesics, non-steroidal anti-inflammatory drugs, mild to moderate opiates (with laxatives if necessary), transcutaneous nerve stimulation, or tricyclic antidepressants. In the most acute cases, in which muscle spasm is severe, one or two doses of diazepam can be useful. Some doctors advocate the use of facet joint injections for diagnostic and therapeutic use.

Rehabilitation involves manual and exercise therapy to mobilise and strengthen the supporting structures of the spine, correction of postural and biomechanical irregularities, and, of course, education of the patient about their back. A multidisciplinary team may need to be involved, particularly when ergonomic issues are thought to be contributing to the pain. Most patients with a prolapsed disc respond to such measures, but surgery may be necessary.

Localised back pain

Spondyloarthropathies

Spondyloarthropathies represent a group of inflammatory arthritides affecting the spine and sacroiliac joints and are associated with iritis, enthesopathies, and variable peripheral arthritis. Included are ankylosing spondylitis, and the reactive, psoriatic, and enteropathic arthritides. The enthesis is the primary site affected, where inflammation is followed by fibrosis and ossification. Features are back and/or buttock pain with morning stiffness. Management depends upon the condition but includes exercise and anti-inflammatory medication.

Spondylolysis and spondylolysthesis

A spondylolysis is a stress fracture through the pars intra-articularis that can be congenital or acquired after repetitive flexion–extension–rotation movements (such as

---

Red flags in the patient with low back pain

- Acute onset in the elderly
- Constant or progressive pain
- Nocturnal pain
- Fever, night sweats, weight loss
- Morning stiffness
- Bilateral or alternating symptoms
- Neurological disturbance
- Sphincter disturbance
- Immunosuppression
- Current or recent infection
- History of malignancy
- Claudicant symptoms, signs of peripheral ischaemia or abdominal mass
- Pain that is not improved with lying in the fetal position or prone with the stomach supported

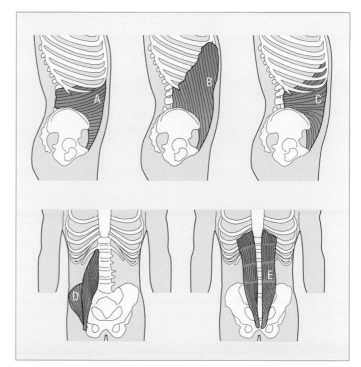

The abdominal muscles are important in the mobility and stability of the lumbar spine. The recti (E=trunk flexion), transversus (A=trunk rotation), and the oblique muscles (B and C=lateral flexion and rotation) are all vital "core stability" muscles that work to stabilise the spine at rest and in movement. Iliopsoas (D) is also an important muscle in spinal and hip stability and movement

---

Patterns of some back disorders

Pain worse with flexion
- Disc prolapse (plus neurological signs)
- Annular tear

Pain worse with extension and rotation
- Facet joint disorder
- Spondylolysis

Localised buttock pain
- Sacroiliac disorder

Claudicant pain eased by flexion
- Spinal stenosis

Progressive bilateral neurological deficit and sphincter disturbance
- Central disc prolapse
- Cauda equina syndrome
- Cord compression
- Spinal vascular accident

occur in bowling during cricket). The lumbosacral region is particularly vulnerable to mechanical stress, because the mobile spine moves on a fixed pelvis in this region, and so lesions are most often seen here. Pain is often localised, is worse with extension and rotation, and may be troublesome at night.

Spondylolisthesis ("vertebral sliding") occurs where bilateral spondylolyses permit vertebral displacement. If displacement is excessive, neurological compromise can occur.

Confirmation of spondylolysis requires oblique radiographs, and a single photon computed tomography scan will show whether the lesion is active.

Treatment of spondylolysis involves relative rest to allow the bone to heal. Bracing can help, but surgery is necessary in a few patients. Persistent pain, progression of the slip, neurological signs, or sphincter disturbance in spondylolysthesis are also indications for surgery.

Annular tears

A decline in water content with age (from 90% in youth to 65% in older patients) reduces the tension in the annulus and contributes to development of tears or fissures in the annulus. As annular tears progress, the nucleus can prolapse through the tear. Acute tears of the annulus can also occur with twisting movements, particularly in flexion.

The sacroiliac joint

The synovial joint is a partially synovial joint bound by many strong ligaments. Pain from the sacroiliac joint can result from a number of causes. Pain thought to arise from the sacroiliac joint can be referred from the lumbar spine.

Sacroiliac joint pain is typically felt in the buttock, but pain may also be felt in the low back or thigh. Lumbar spine extension often exacerbates symptoms, but clinical tests lack specificity. A bone scan with sacroiliac indices is indicated if sacroiliitis is suspected. Management depends on the cause. Relative rest, anti-inflammatories, or rarely a fluoroscopic guided steroid injection may all be indicated for pain control.

The figure showing the abdominal muscles is adapted from Norris C. *Abdominal training: nutrition and fitness.* London: A&C Black, 1997

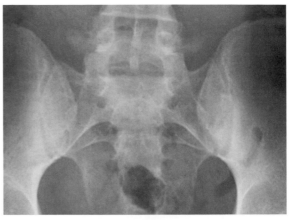

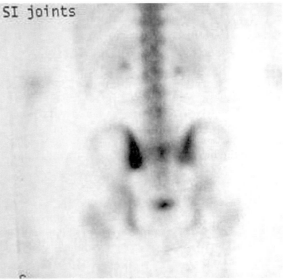

Plain x ray radiograph and corresponding bone scan in sacroiliitis

---

Causes of sacroiliac pain

- Inflammation (sacroiliitis)
  Seronegative arthritis
  Infection
- Major trauma
- Stress fractures across the joint
- Mechanical stresses (sports people)

Further reading

Epidemiology
- Waddell G, ed. *Epidemiology review: the epidemiology and cost of back pain.* London: Stationery Office, 1994
- Croft P, Stevens A, Rafferty J. *Health care needs assessment: low back pain.* Oxford: Radcliffe Medical Press, 1997

Imaging
- Royal College of Radiologists. *Making the best use of department of clinical radiology: guidelines for doctors.* London: Royal College of Radiologists, 1999

Management
- van Tulder M, Koes B. Low back pain and sciatica: acute. *Clin Evid* 2002;7:1018-31
- van Tulder M, Koes B. Low back pain and sciatica: chronic. *Clin Evid* 2002;7:1032-48
- Managing acute low back pain. *Drug Ther Bull* 1998;36:93-95
- Philadelphia Panel. Philadelphia Panel evidence-based clinical practice guidelines on selected rehabilitation interventions for low back pain *Phys Ther* 2001;81:1641-74 (www.rcgp.org.uk/rcgp/clinspec/guidelines/backpain/index.asp)

5 Pain in the hip and knee

Andrew J Hamer

Pain in the hip

Childhood
A child with hip disease may not present with pain or a history of trauma but with an unexplained limp. Unexplained knee pain should raise the suspicion of hip abnormality.

Congenital dislocation of the hip
Ultrasound screening should detect at risk cases, but missed cases may present as a delay in walking, limp, or discrepancy in leg length. Children usually present before five years of age. Missed cases may lead to a non-congruent joint and early osteoarthritic degeneration in adulthood.

Perthes disease
Disintegration of the femoral head, with subsequent healing and deformity of the hip, usually occurs in boys aged 5-10 years. The precise cause is unclear, but segmental avascular necrosis of the femoral head is probably responsible. A limp, hip pain, or knee pain may result. Treatment aims to contain the femoral head in the acetabulum to reduce the risks of future osteoarthritis.

Slipped upper femoral epiphysis
This condition is typically seen in overweight, hypogonadal boys, who often present with pain referred to the knee, although girls are not immune from the condition. The diagnosis may be difficult, but a "frog lateral" x ray radiograph will show the deformity.

Surgical stabilisation is needed as a matter of urgency to prevent further slippage of the epiphysis. The contralateral hip is at high risk of slippage, and patients and parents should be warned to return if any knee or hip pain occurs.

Septic arthritis
This is relatively uncommon, but it should be suspected in a child who is ill, toxic, and unable to walk. Movement of the affected joint is not possible because of pain. Diagnosis is confirmed by raised white cell count and erythrocyte sedimentation rate and perhaps by effusion on ultrasound images. Urgent surgical drainage is vital to reduce the risk of late osteoarthritis. Diagnosis may be particularly difficult in neonates. *Staphylococcus aureus* is the usual infective organism.

Transient synovitis or "irritable hip"
A reactive effusion may occur in the hip in association with a systemic viral illness. Affected children are not acutely unwell and can move the hip, but with some degree of stiffness. An effusion may be seen on ultrasound images and the condition is usually self-limiting. Perthes' disease may present in the early stages with an effusion without changes visible on x ray examination.

Other arthritides
Juvenile chronic arthritis may present with hip pain. General management of the arthritic process is important, with physiotherapy to prevent joint contracture.

Important causes of childhood hip pain
- Congenital dislocation of the hip
- Perthes disease
- Slipped upper femoral epiphysis
- Septic arthritis
- Transient synovitis or "irritable hip"
- Other arthritides

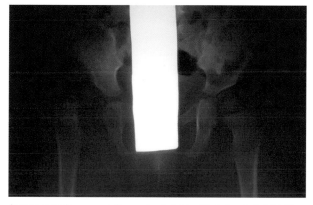

Anteroposterior x ray radiograph of child with dislocated right hip. Note the lateral displacement of the femur and the poorly developed ossific nucleus of the hip

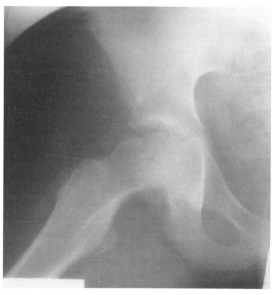

X ray radiograph of a child's right hip. Displacement of the epiphysis relative to the femoral neck is easily seen

Adults

Pain from the hip is usually felt in the groin or lateral or anterior thigh. Referred pain to the knee often catches out the unwary! Although buttock pain may originate from the hip, the lumbar spine is the usual source. Hip disorders often produce a limp, a reduction in the distance that can be walked, and stiffness, which prevents activities of daily living, such as getting in and out of baths, putting on shoes, and foot care.

Osteoarthritis

Osteoarthritis is one of the most common causes of hip pain in adults; although usually seen in their 60s, it can present at any age. Rest, simple analgesia, or a walking stick often relieve the pain. A limp may develop, with associated stiffness. In extreme situations, leg length is lost, and the hip adopts a fixed flexion and adduction deformity. Total hip replacement is extremely effective at relieving pain in osteoarthritis.

Other arthritides

Rheumatoid arthritis, psoriatic arthritis, and ankylosing spondylitis can also produce hip pain. The last is particularly associated with stiffness. Total hip replacement is often needed.

Hip fracture

Osteoporotic hip fracture in elderly women is epidemic. A fall followed by inability to bear weight and a short externally rotated leg are diagnostic. An undisplaced fracture may not stop the patient bearing weight, and it may not be visible on initial x ray examination. Repeat films are usually required, and a bone scan or magnetic resonance imaging if there is doubt. Treatment is by surgical stabilisation or by replacement of the femoral head (hemiarthroplasty). Considerable comorbidity is often found.

Paget's disease

The pelvis is often involved in Paget's disease, and can cause hip pain. Treatment of the disease with bisphosphonates can reduce pain, but co-existent osteoarthritis of the hip can also occur.

Avascular necrosis

Segmental avascular necrosis of the weight-bearing portion of the femoral head can occur. This produces progressive pain, limp, and late secondary osteoarthritis. Magnetic resonance imaging gives a diagnosis in the early stages, but if radiological evidence is established, surgical treatment to arrest the disease is less successful. Hip replacement may ultimately be required.

Malignancy

Metastases in the pelvis or proximal femur will produce hip pain. Treatment with local radiotherapy or bisphosphonates, or both, may slow the disease progress. Surgical stabilisation of impending fractures may be required. Primary bone tumours as a cause of hip pain are extremely rare.

Infection

Primary septic arthritis is rare in adults, but it may present insidiously in immunocompromised patients. Plain x ray examinations and ultrasound scanning may be needed to show the presence of an effusion. Surgical drainage is usually necessary.

Painful soft tissue conditions around the hip

Trochanteric bursitis—This is usually self-limiting inflammation of the bursa between the greater trochanter and fascia lata. It is characterised by pain over the trochanter (not in the groin) and local physiotherapy, anti-inflammatories, rest,

---

Causes of hip pain in adults

- Osteoarthritis
- Other arthritides
    Rheumatoid arthritis
    Psoriatic arthritis
    Ankylosing spondylitis
- Hip fracture
- Paget's disease
- Avascular necrosis
- Malignancy
- Infection
- Painful soft tissue conditions around the hip
    Trochanteric bursitis
    Snapping ilio-psoas tendon
    Torn acetabular labrum

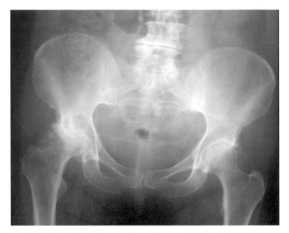

Osteoarthritis of the right hip, with joint space loss, subarticular cysts, peripheral osteophytes, and subchondral sclerosis

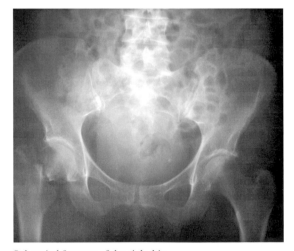

Subcapital fracture of the right hip

Causes of avascular necrosis

- Most cases are idiopathic
- Associated conditions include:
    Excess alcohol
    Prolonged steroid therapy
    Working in pressurised environments
    (for example, deep sea divers)

and occasionally local anaesthetic and steroid injections can help.

Snapping ilio-psoas tendon—This causes a painful "clunk" in the groin when the hip goes from extension to flexion. The hip is otherwise normal. The psoas tendon impinges on the capsule of the hip anteriorally to produce discomfort. Diagnosis is made if movement of fluoroscopic x ray contrast agent injected into the psoas tendon is abnormal. Surgical release may be needed.

Torn acetabular labrum—This produces pain in the groin on rotatory movements of the hip, and the hip may feel unstable or give way. Magnetic resonance imaging shows the abnormality, and the torn labrum can be removed arthroscopically.

Knee pain

Knee pain may present spontaneously or after injury. Stiffness or the inability to extend the knee fully indicate effusion within the joint. An effusion can be detected by the disappearance of the dimples either side of the patella, and it may produce a patellar "tap", in which the patella can be pushed onto the anterior surface of the femur by the examiner's fingers.

Knee pain may be referred from the hip (see slipped upper femoral epiphysis, above). The knee is a much more superficial joint than the hip, and so the site of pain and tenderness often indicates the site of an abnormality.

Children
Anterior knee pain
Seen in adolescent girls, this is often named chondromalacia patellae, which implies softening of cartilage on the posterior aspect of the patella. Pain usually settles at skeletal maturity.

Patella subluxation
Seen in girls with patellar maltracking, this is sometimes related to tibial torsional deformities or valgus knees. It usually responds to physiotherapy.

Osgood-Schlatter disease
This is an osteochondritis of the tibial tubercle seen in adolescent boys. Localised pain and tenderness, and swelling of the insertion of the patellar tendon are seen. Appropriate analgesia only is required, as the condition is self-limiting.

Adults
Knee injuries
Sporting injuries of the knees often occur. A twisting injury during football, with sudden pain, swelling of the whole knee, and problems bearing weight indicate haemarthrosis. This may be due to a torn cruciate ligament or major meniscal detachment. A slowly developing effusion after a similar injury suggests a smaller meniscal tear.

A valgus strain to the knee may tear the medial collateral ligament, which produces medial pain and tenderness but no effusion. Falls from heights and significant traumas can produce intra-articular knee fractures that need urgent orthopaedic referral.

Spontaneous knee pain, redness, and swelling
Acute arthritis may produce significant swelling, heat, and pain in the knee. Septic arthritis should be excluded if the patient is systemically unwell, although the signs can be masked by steroid therapy.

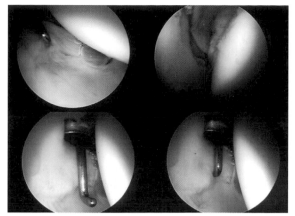

Arthroscopic images of a hip. Top left: Shows small acetabular labral tear

> **Always examine the hip in a child with knee pain**

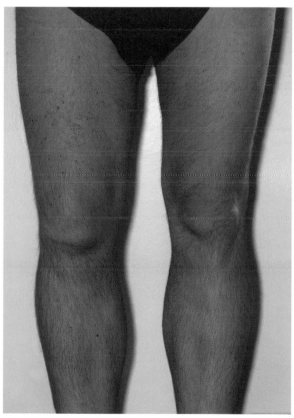

Right knee effusion. Note the loss of the "dimples" either side of the patella in comparison with the left knee

> **Intra-articular steroids should never be given until sepsis has been excluded**

The knee should be aspirated under aseptic conditions and the fluid cultured to establish the diagnosis. Examination of the fluid for crystals should also be carried out.

Gout, pseudogout, or other types of arthritis such as Reiter's syndrome, can all produce an acute, hot, red knee.

Chronic pain and swelling

Osteoarthritis in the knee usually affects the medial compartment, with the development of a typical varus deformity. An effusion may be present, with medial joint line tenderness. Rheumatoid arthritis produces synovitis and effusions but may lead to a valgus deformity. Both may need total knee arthroplasty if conservative measures fail. Other arthritides, such as ankylosing spondylitis and psoriatic arthritis, may affect the knees.

Chronic pain and instability

Recurrent medial joint line pain, instability, and tenderness may indicate a chronic medial meniscal tear, or osteoarthritis. Loose bodies may be produced in osteoarthritis, which can cause instability and intermittent pain, and may be palpable if they lie in the suprapatellar pouch. Osteochondritis dissecans is characterised by separation of areas of articular cartilage from their bony bed, leading to pain, swelling, and the knee "giving way." The loose bodies may be palpable. Typical sites for such separation include the medial femoral condyle and the patella. A chronically unstable knee may indicate an old anterior cruciate ligament rupture. Surgery is only indicated for significant instability and perhaps in professional sportspeople.

Localised pain and swelling

Bursae occur in several sites around the knee. Swelling over the patellar ligament occurs with chronic kneeling; it responds to appropriate knee pads. Popliteal cysts ("Baker's cysts") usually reflect underlying knee pathology and respond to treatment of the synovitis. Removal is potentially hazardous, and recurrence is common.

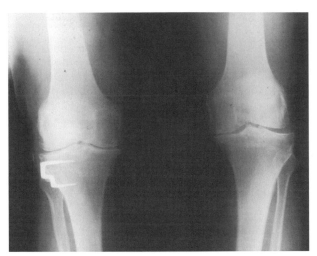

Osteoarthritis of both knees. The left shows typical medial compartment disease, the right shows medial and lateral disease. The patient has previously had a high tibial osteotomy

Semimembranous bursae are common in children, on the posteromedial aspect of the knee. They usually disappear as the child grows

Further reading

- Solomon L, Nayagam D, Warwick D. *Apley's System of Orthopaedics and Fractures.* 8th ed. London: Arnold, 2001
- McRae R. *Clinical Orthopaedic Examination.* Edinburgh: Churchill Livingstone, 1997
- Miller MD, ed. *Review of Orthopaedics.* Philadelphia: WB Saunders, 2000

6 Pain in the foot

James Woodburn, Philip S Helliwell

Foot pain is common. It may be caused by local disease, be associated with systemic disease, or be a reflection of chronic widespread pain. In general, a multidisciplinary approach to treatment is preferable. This is reflected in increasingly close liaison between podiatry, rheumatology, and orthopaedic departments. State registered podiatrists offer a range of treatments from skin lesion care to orthoses and, more recently, ambulatory forefoot surgery. To understand dysfunction, clinicians should be familiar with the normal development and anatomical variants of the foot.

Pain in children

Pain may be associated with congenital abnormalities such as equino-varus deformity. Such structural abnormalities may reflect underlying neurological diseases, such as cerebral palsy. A rigid pronated foot in the early teens may be the first symptom of a tarsal coalition. Gait abnormalities, such as intoeing, may be of concern to parents, but they are seldom treated actively.

Juvenile chronic arthritis

The knee and ankle joints are most often affected in all subtypes of juvenile chronic arthritis. Children may present with a limp or reluctance to walk. In the hind foot, pain and reflex muscle spasm can lead to valgus deformity (in two thirds of cases) or varus deformity (in one third of cases). In some patients, this may progress to bony ankylosis. The child may be reluctant to push off with the forefoot during walking, and pressure studies show poor contact of the foot to the floor. Lack of use can lead to delayed maturation of bone or soft tissue, and, in such cases, discrepancy in leg length should be sought carefully.

Pain in the forefoot (metatarsalgia)

Morton's metatarsalgia (interdigital neuroma)

This normally affects the proximal part of the plantar digital nerve and accompanying plantar digital artery. Trauma to these structures leads to histological changes, including inflammatory oedema, microscopic changes in the neurolemma, fibrosis, and, later, degeneration of the nerve. Morton's neuroma is the result of an entrapment lesion of the interdigital nerve.

Clinical features

Clinical features include a gradual onset, with sudden attacks of neuralgic pain or paraesthesia during walking—often in the third and fourth toe. Examination may show lesser toe deformities, slight splaying of the forefoot, abnormal pronation, and hallux valgus. These often occur in women who wear court shoes. Compression of the cleft or laterally across the metatarsal heads may produce acute pain and the characteristic "Mulder's click."

Characteristics of the adult foot

Three main types of foot
- Normal
- Pronated (flat)
- Supinated (high arch)

Examination
- **Examine** the foot when bearing weight and when unloaded
- **Inspect** patient's shoes for abnormal or uneven wear
- **Consult** a podiatrist if a structural or mechanical abnormality is suspected—many can be treated with orthoses

---

Characteristics of children's feet

Normal foot
- Flexible foot structure (may look flat with a valgus heel)
- Medial longitudinal arch forms when child stands on tiptoe
- Heel to toe walking
- Forefoot in line with rear foot
- Mobile joints with painless motion and no swelling
- Adopts adult morphology by about eight years of age

Abnormal foot
- Inflexible
- Lesser toe deformities
- Rigid valgus (pronated) foot with everted heel position
- High arch foot with toe retraction and tight extensor tendons
- Toe walking
- Delay or difficulty in walking or running
- Abducted or adducted forefoot relative to heel
- Pain, swelling, or stiffness of joints
- Hallux deformity

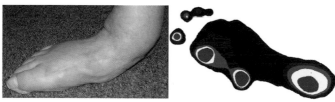

Abnormally pronated foot, with pressure profile showing large weight-bearing surface and higher pressures medially

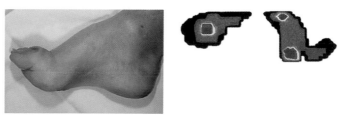

Abnormally supinated foot, with pressure profile showing small weight-bearing surface and high pressures over first and fifth metatarsal heads

Treatment

Patients should be given advice about suitable footwear and possibly should be given orthoses to control abnormal pronation. Injections of local anaesthetic and hydrocortisone around the nerve, or surgical excision, can be helpful.

Stress fracture (march fracture)

Stress fractures are associated with increased activity, and lesions can affect any of the metatarsal shafts, often along the line of the surgical neck. They can occasionally be seen in patients with osteoporosis as a pathological fracture.

Clinical features

Patients have a history of a change in the amount of activity, change in occupation or footwear, or sudden weight gain. The symptom is a dull ache along the affected metatarsal shaft, which changes to a sharp ache just behind the metatarsal head. The pain is exacerbated by exercise and is more acute at "toe off." Tenderness and swelling is felt over the dorsal surface of the shaft. Pain is produced by compression of the metatarsal head or traction of the toe. X ray examination may not show the fracture for 2-4 weeks, but if it is important to confirm the diagnosis—for example, for an athlete who needs advice on whether to continue playing sport—a bone scan can reveal it earlier.

Treatment

Rest and local protective padding with partial immobilisation are usually enough. These fractures rarely require casting.

Acute synovitis

This condition is normally associated with acute trauma, which leads to inflammation of the synovial membrane and effusion. Systemic causes of acute synovitis, such as rheumatoid arthritis or infection, should be excluded when making a diagnosis.

Clinical features

It is rare in children but often affects young adults. Patients complain of a sudden onset of painful throbbing that is made worse by movement. The patient may have experienced trauma or have a systemic inflammatory disorder. Any movement of the joint produces pain. Fusiform swelling is present around the distended joint, and crepitus may be felt.

Treatment

Rest, immobilisation, and ultrasound treatment may help if trauma is the cause. Anti-inflammatory drugs sometimes help. Previously unsuspected systemic arthritis should be investigated.

Acute inflammation of anterior metatarsal soft tissue pad

This common condition is generally found in middle-aged women. It affects the soft tissues of the plantar aspect of the forefoot and is associated with increased shear forces, such as occur when wearing "slip on" and high-heeled court shoes.

Clinical features

Patients present with a burning or throbbing pain localised to the soft tissues anterior to the metatarsal heads. The pain usually develops over a few weeks, is often associated with walking in a particular pair of shoes, and is usually relieved by rest. The tissues are inflamed, warm, and congested. Direct palpation, rotation, and simulation of shear forces on the foot

---

Causes of pain in the fore foot

Primary
- Functional and structural forefoot pathologies

Secondary
- Rheumatoid disease
- Stress lesions
- Post-traumatic syndromes
- Diabetes
- Gout
- Paralytic deformity
- Sesamoid pathology
- Osteoarthritis

Unrelated to weight distribution
- Nerve root pathology
- Tarsal tunnel nerve compression syndrome
    Analogous to carpal tunnel syndrome
    Often misdiagnosed as foot strain or plantar fasciitis
    Primary symptom is burning feeling on sole of foot in the dermatome served by the medial plantar nerve

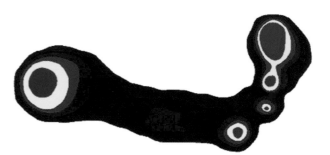

Pressure profile of the right foot of a 54-year-old patient with rheumatoid arthritis. Note absent lesser toe contact and high pressure (hot colours) over central metatarsal heads

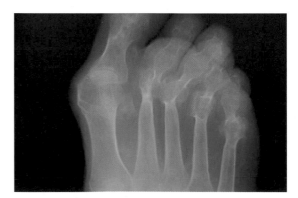

Advanced destruction in the forefoot of a patient with rheumatoid arthritis

exacerbate the pain. Examination of patients' shoes may reveal a worn insole, with a depression under the metatarsal heads.

Management
Advice on footwear, with adequate support or cushioning, should be given. Associated abnormal pronation or lesser toe deformities should be corrected with orthoses.

Osteochondritis (Freiberg's infraction)
This quite common condition generally affects the second or third metatarsal heads. It is an aseptic necrosis or epiphyseal infraction associated with trauma and localised minute thrombosis of the epiphysis.

Clinical features
Osteochondritis affects teenagers and is associated with increased sporting activity. The presenting complaint is often a limp, with dull pain associated with movement of the metatarsal phalangeal joint, exacerbated at toe off. The long-term result is a flattened metatarsal head, which can progress to arthritis. The affected joint may be slightly swollen, with a disparity in toe length and width. Traction causes pain. Restricted movement may be due to muscle spasm in the early stages and later to arthritis. Radiographs show distortion of the metatarsal head.

Treatment
In the early stages, rest and immobilisation are enough, but sometimes patients eventually need corrective surgery.

Plantar metatarsal bursitis
This condition may affect the deep anatomical or superficial adventitious bursae. In the acute form—such as in dancers, squash players, or skiers—the first metatarsal is usually affected, while the second to fourth metatarsals are affected in chronic inflammatory arthritis.

Clinical features
Patients present with a throbbing pain under a metatarsal head that usually persists at rest and is exacerbated when the area is first loaded. The acute condition affects men and women equally, usually in younger adults. If a superficial bursa is affected there will be signs of acute inflammation, with fluctuant swelling and warmth. With deep bursitis, the tissues are tight and congested. Direct pressure or compression produces pain, as does dorsiflexion of the associated digit.

Treatment
Anti-inflammatory drugs are useful; in practice, local gels and systemic oral drugs help. Injections of corticosteroid may be indicated in severe cases. Patients must rest the affected part; this may be achieved by protective padding. Any underlying deformity or foot type with abnormal function should be assessed and treated.

Plantar fascia affections

Pain along the medial longitudinal arch is quite common. Most affected patients have abnormal foot mechanics, such as abnormal pronation, valgus heel, or a flat foot. Mechanical dysfunction and change in medial arch posture can place strain on soft tissues, which results in localised or more diffuse pain—the foot's equivalent to "low back pain" syndrome. Other conditions include true plantar fasciitis, which is characterised by a few fast growing nodules in the fascia, and plantar

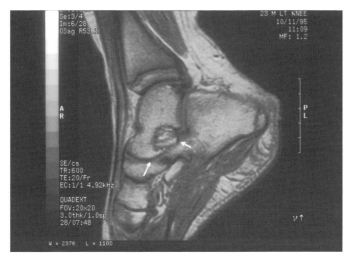
Tarsal coalition. Magnetic resonance image in a patient with calcaneonavicular coalition. Note synostosis between the calcaneus and navicular bones (arrows)

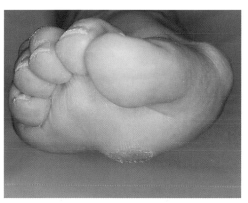
Severe plantar metatarsal bursitis affecting second metatarsal head of patient with rheumatoid arthritis. Overlying callus suggests that this is a high pressure site during normal gait

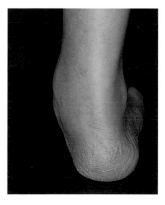
Valgus heel with bulging of the talar head medially

fibromatosis, which is characterised by fibrous nodules and contracture of the fascia.

Treatment of true plantar fascial strain requires rest and control of abnormal function with orthoses. Ultrasound treatment seems helpful, but controlled trials are lacking.

Painful heel

Sever's disease (calcaneal apophysitis)
This was thought to be an avascular necrosis of growing bone but is now interpreted as a chronic strain at the attachment of the posterior apophysis of the calcaneus to the main body of the bone, possibly from pull of the Achilles tendon. It therefore is analogous to Osgood-Schlatter disease of the tibial tuberosity.

Clinical features
The condition usually affects boys aged 8-13 years, who complain of a dull ache behind the heel of gradual onset that is exacerbated by jumping or occurs just before heel lift. A limp is usually seen with early heel lift. Rest normally relieves the pain. Tenderness is seen over the lower posterior part of the tuberosity of the calcaneus. Radiographs are usually normal.

Treatment
In most cases, reassurance and advice about reducing activities will suffice: the condition usually subsides spontaneously. In some cases, heel lifts help; occasionally, if the pain is severe, a below knee walking cast is needed.

Plantar calcaneal bursitis (policeman's heel)
This is inflammation of the adventitious bursa beneath the plantar aspect of the calcaneal tuberosities. It is associated with shearing stress caused by an altered angle of heel strike.

Clinical features
The condition is characterised by an increasingly severe burning, aching, and throbbing pain on the plantar surface of the heel. A history of increased activity or weight gain is usual. The heel seems normal but may feel warm. Direct pressure or sideways compression causes pain. The tissues may feel tight and congested.

Treatment
Rest and local anti-inflammatory drugs may be useful. Heel cushions and medial arch supports are also used. Little evidence supports ultrasound treatment or shortwave diathermy.

Chronic inflammation of the heel pad
This is a distinct clinical condition that usually results from trauma or heavy heel strike. It sometimes is seen in elderly people as their fat pads atrophy or in those who suddenly become more active.

Clinical features
A generalised warm dull throbbing pain is felt over the weight-bearing area of the heel; this develops over a few months. The pain is most intense typically on first rising. Tenderness is experienced over the heel, which feels tight and distended.

Treatment
Normally, this condition improves with time and rest. Soft heel cushions and medial arch fillers sometimes help. Ultrasound treatment and short wave diathermy are often used, but

---

Common causes of painful heel
Pain within heel
- Disease of calcaneus-osteomyelitis, tumours, Paget's disease
- Arthritis of subtalar joint complex

Pain behind heel
- Haglund's deformity ("pump bumps," "heel bumps")
- Rupture of Achilles tendon
- Achilles paratendinitis
- Posterior tibial paratendinitis or tenosynovitis
- Peroneal paratendinitis or tenosynovitis
- Posterior calcaneal bursitis
- Calcaneal apophysitis

Pain beneath heel
- Tender heel pad
- Plantar fasciitis

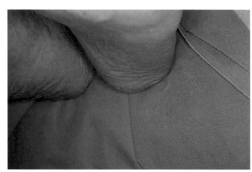

Chronic painful plantar heel bursitis

Achilles tendon affections
Tendinitis
- Presents as painful local swelling of tendon, which moves with the tendon as the foot is dorsiflexed and plantar flexed
- Important to check tendon for evidence of partial or complete rupture, which is often missed because of inflammation

Peritendinitis
- Presents as large diffuse swelling of tissues surrounding tendon, which remains static as the tendon is stretched.
- Patients experience pain and crepitus on palpation

Achilles tendon bursitis
- Presents as diffuse fusiform swelling inferior to Achilles tendon, which fills the normal indentation seen below the malleoli and deep to the Achilles tendon

controlled trials are few. Steroid injections have an early effect but do not influence the condition's favourable natural history. Steroid injections can be more painful than the condition unless they are done carefully, with adequate slow infiltration of local anaesthetic (or an ankle tibial nerve block) before injection.

Achilles tendon affections

Inflammation of the Achilles tendon and surrounding soft tissue may be associated with overuse or systemic inflammatory disorders. Inflammation of the tendon, peritendon tissues, and bursae give slightly different clinical pictures. Conditions such as xanthoma can also affect the Achilles tendon and produce fusiform swelling in the tendon. In such cases, cholesterol concentrations should be checked and treated if raised.

Clinical features

Clinical features vary according to the tissues affected. Increased activity leading to an overuse syndrome may be a feature in younger active patients.

Treatment

Treatment depends on the primary cause. Partial or complete ruptures of the tendon need immobilisation and surgical repair. For inflammatory conditions, non-steroidal anti-inflammatory drugs may help, as may ultrasound treatment, friction, rest, and shock-absorbing heel lifts. Inflammation may be triggered by overuse through poor foot mechanics; in such cases, orthoses may control the pronation. Hydrocortisone injections may be useful if the bursa or peritendons are affected, but they are contraindicated for the tendon itself. Ultrasound imaging may be useful.

Arthropathies that affect the foot

Osteoarthritis

Osteoarthritis in the foot may be asymptomatic, but it can lead to pain, joint stiffness, functional loss, and disability. The most common sites are the first metatarsophalangeal joint (hallux rigidus) and the tarsus joints. Biomechanical factors are often involved in the development of degenerative joint changes (for example, compensatory foot pronation in subtalar osteoarthritis). Trauma, recurrent urate gout, and the demands of fashion—such as inappropriate footwear—are other factors; however, the broad style of modern shoes may be beneficial.

Rheumatoid arthritis

Rheumatoid arthritis often starts in the foot, particularly at the metatarsophalangeal joints. The forefoot is painful and stiff,

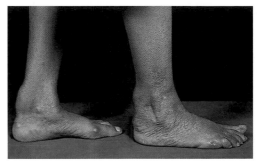

Chronic inflammation of Achilles tendon is another cause of heel pain. This should not be treated by local injection of corticosteroid

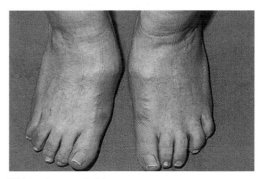

Midtarsal osteoarthritis

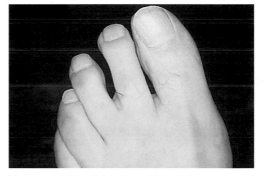

Metatarsophalangeal joint synovitis in early rheumatoid arthritis: note a widening of the first and second cleft—the "daylight sign"

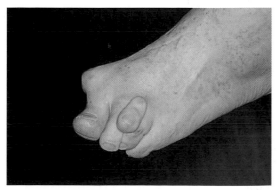

Extensive foot deformity

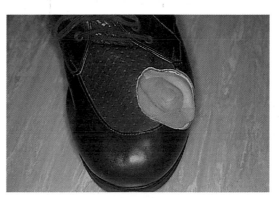

Drastic self-adjustment of surgical shoes to gain pain relief

and direct transverse pressure to the forefoot or squeezing a single metatarsophalangeal joint is painful. Non-specific metatarsalgia is often diagnosed. In the early stages of the disease, the hindfoot, particularly the subtalar joint, may also be painful. Synovitis of tendon sheaths around the ankle may also occur. In chronic rheumatoid feet, severe pain in the forefoot may continue, with a sensation of walking on pebbles. Gross deformity causes dysfunction and disability.

Seronegative spondyloarthritis

This group includes ankylosing spondylitis, psoriatic arthritis, undifferentiated seronegative arthropathy, and reactive arthritis. Achilles peritendinitis, and retrocalcaneal bursitis can be seen. In radiographs, inflammatory spurs may be seen on the calcaneum at the insertion points of the Achilles tendon and plantar fascia. Asymmetrical heel pain may result from a plantar calcaneal enthesopathy.

The pattern of articular involvement in the foot may vary from a single "sausage toe" (dactylitis) to a very destructive arthritis. Painful stiff interphalangeal and metatarsophalangeal joints, often in an asymmetrical pattern, are common. Claw toe and hallux valgus deformity are more obvious. Nail dystrophy may be seen, with typical psoriatic pitting, onycholysis, subungual hyperkeratosis, discoloration, and transverse ridging.

Pustular psoriasis and keratoderma blennorrhagica on the plantar aspect of the foot may contribute to pain when walking.

Gout

Chapter 9 discusses the manifestations of acute gout in the foot. In the chronic state, tophi in the foot may ulcerate if they act as pressure points. Permanent destructive joint damage and deformity may result and lead to painful dysfunction in the foot.

Management of rheumatic foot conditions

Patients with rheumatic foot problems are best managed by a team that includes a physician, a surgeon, and therapists. Podiatrists have a particular role in several aspects of care.

Common abnormalities in the rheumatoid foot

- Hallux valgus
- Lesser toe deformities—for example, hammer toes and claw toes
- Prominent metatarsal heads with overlying painful callosities or ulceration
- Pronation of foot with valgus heel deformity and collapse of midtarsal joint, giving a flatfooted appearance
- Tenosynovitis, especially of tibialis posterior and peroneal tendons, plantar heel bursitis, calcaneal spur, and tendoachilles bursitis
- Tarsal tunnel nerve compression syndrome

Tissue viability
Joint deformity causes pressure lesions such as callosities, corns, or ulceration and may be compounded by other factors such as ingrowing toe nails, peripheral neuropathy, or the effects of systemic corticosteroids. Podiatrists undertake procedures such as scalpel reduction, design and manufacture of insoles and orthoses, and surgery under local anaesthesia to relieve pain and restore or maintain tissue viability.

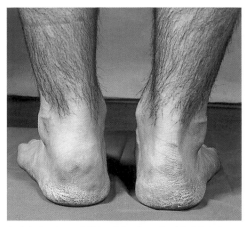

Ankylosing spondylitis of the feet: the hind foot is predominantly affected

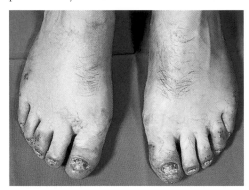

Psoriatic arthropathy

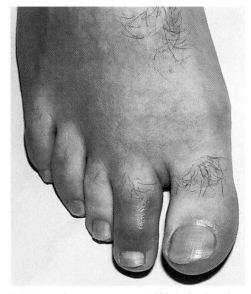

Reiter's syndrome—sausage toe (this is also found with psoriatic arthropathy)

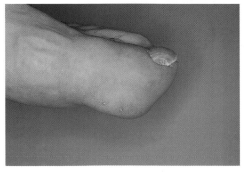

Large painful tophi over the interphalangeal joint of the hallux

Foot function and joint protection

Foot dysfunction due to arthritis can be improved with orthoses, which can be ready made or individually designed from casts. Orthoses may be used to control deformities—such as the valgus heel seen in rheumatoid arthritis—but they also have a major role in maintaining tissue viability and relieving pain (be it joint, soft tissue, or skin lesion in origin). Training towards gait modification may be necessary, and pressure-relieving orthoses of a total contact design may serve to reduce pressures at painful joint sites.

Foot health promotion

Patients will often need advice on daily care of feet. Family members may be involved when patients cannot reach their feet or are unable to perform tasks on the feet because of other disability. Advice may be needed on splints, walking aids, footwear, insoles, foot hygiene, and exercise.

Foot surgery

Foot surgery may be effective for relieving pain and improving deformity when conservative measures have failed. Many rheumatic patients have conditions of the toenails that need surgery under local anaesthetic; they are best dealt with by an experienced clinician such as a podiatrist.

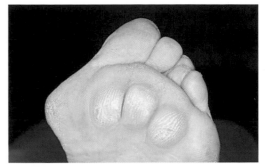
"Walking on pebbles"—metatarsophalangeal callosities in rheumatoid arthritis

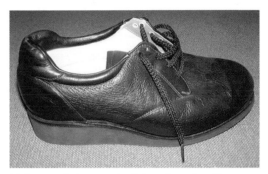
Modern stock shoes can be light and comfortable

Use of orthoses for rheumatic foot problems needs suitable footwear; podiatrists and orthotists should liaise when extra depth shoes or surgical shoes are needed

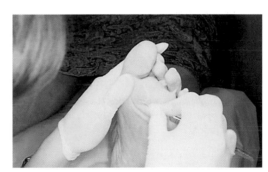
Scalpel debridement of plantar lesions provides effective pain relief

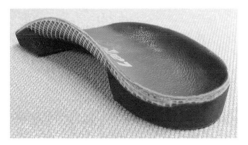
Custom-made rigid orthoses act as splints to support inflamed joints in early rheumatoid arthritis

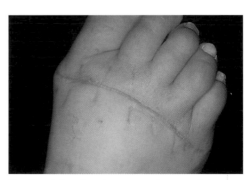
Forefoot arthroplasty is necessary in cases of severe fore foot pain and deformity

Further reading

- Fam AG. The ankle and foot: regional pain problems. In: Klippel JH, Dieppe PA, eds. *Rheumatology*. London: Mosby, 1998:4/12.1-4/12.12
- Jayson MIV, Smidt LA, eds. *The foot in arthritis*. London: Baillière Tindall, 1987
- Hintermann B, Nigg BM, Hames MR, Cooper PS, Sammarco GJ, Renstrom PAFH, et al. Foot and ankle. In: Nordin M, Anderson GBJ, Pope MH, eds. *Musculoskeletal disorders in the workplace: principles and practice*. St Louis: Mosby, 1997:537-95
- Rana NA. Rheumatoid arthritis, other collagen diseases, and psoriasis of the foot. In: Jahss MH, ed. *Disorders of the foot and ankle: medical and surgical management*. Philadelphia: WB Saunders, 1991:1719-51
- Woodburn J, Helliwell PS. Foot problems in rheumatology. *Br J Rheumatol* 1997;36:932-4

7 Fibromyalgia: musculoskeletal distress

Sarah Ryan, Anne Browne

Fibromyalgia syndrome is used to describe widespread musculoskeletal pain and hyperalgesic tender spots with no identified organic cause. Although the term fibromyalgia is not ideal, it focuses attention on the main symptom: generalised allodynia or hyperalgesia. The pain is often accompanied by stiffness and non-restorative sleep. Additional physical and psychological associations are often present. That patients have a greater lifetime frequency of depression is well documented. The varied presentation and heterogeneity of the condition is recognised, and diagnosis is hampered by the absence of objective clinical indicators. Studies show that the symptoms persist over time, with continuing functional impairment and high use of health services.

Fibromyalgia is one of the most common conditions seen in outpatient rheumatology clinics. In North America, 20% of referrals to rheumatologists relate to fibromyalgia, and 2% of people in population studies have symptoms compatible with a diagnosis of fibromyalgia.

Diagnosis

The American College of Rheumatology originated criteria for the classification of fibromyalgia for research purposes. Although this definition provides guidance, the diagnosis of fibromyalgia is clinical and, in practice, patients may present with fewer than 11 of the designated tender spots but still be diagnosed with fibromyalgia. The reliability of the tender joint count as a reflection of clinical status has been questioned. Physical examination excludes systemic illness, inflammatory arthritis, muscle weakness, and neurological abnormalities. Reported symptoms and objective findings are often in discordance. Clinical findings are unremarkable, and the doctor's main finding is the presence of multiple hyperalgesic tender sites. In healthy people, such sites are uncomfortable to firm pressure, but in patients with fibromyalgia, the same pressure elicits a wince or withdrawal response. Non-tender sites can be used as control sites. Limited haematological and biochemical screenings (for example, thyroid function tests, full blood count, biochemical profile, and inflammatory markers) will exclude other causes for the symptoms, including polymyalgia rheumatica, inflammatory spondyloarthropathy, and hypothyroidism, as such tests are normal in fibromyalgia.

Other symptoms (headaches, dizziness, and paraesthaesia), have often been investigated extensively, with no cause found. Fibromyalgia may superimpose on pre-existing painful conditions, such as osteoarthritis, but it usually affects people with no other diagnosis. Unless evidence suggests an associated arthritis or cervical or lumbar radiculopathy, radiological investigations are not indicated clinically. Unnecessary tests should be avoided, as the management approach focuses on a biopsychosocial perspective and self-management strategies.

Clinical picture

The typical patient (if such a person exists) is a female in her third or fourth decade of life, with a history of longstanding

---

Physical and psychological associations with fibromyalgia

Physical
- Irritable bladder
- Irritable bowel
- Migraines
- Muscle spasms
- Dizziness
- Perceptions of swelling
- Paraesthaesia
- Temperature changes

Psychological
- Panic attacks
- Anxiety
- Depression
- Irritability
- Memory lapses
- Word mix ups
- Reduced concentration

American College of Rheumatology's definition of fibromyalgia (1990)

- History of widespread musculoskeletal pain in all four quadrants of body, plus axial pain (cervical spine, anterior chest, thoracic spine, or low back)
- Duration of pain at least three months
- Multiple hyperalgesic tender spots determined by digital palpation using firm pressure (equal to force of 4 kg) in 11 of 18 tender spots. Hyperalgesia absent at normally non-tender sites; these areas can be used as control sites, that is forehead, thumbnail, and distal forearm
- Sites all bilateral and situated in: Suboccipital muscle insertions (posterior base of skull)
  Low cervical spine (C4-C6 interspinous ligaments)
  Low lumbar spine (L4-S1 interspinous ligament)
  Midpoint of upper trapezius
  Origins of supraspinatus muscle above scapula spines
  Second costochondral junctions, on upper surface lateral to junctions
  Two centimetres distal to lateral epicondyles
  In upper outer quadrants of buttocks in anterior fold of gluteus medius
  Greater trochanter
  Medial fat pad of knee

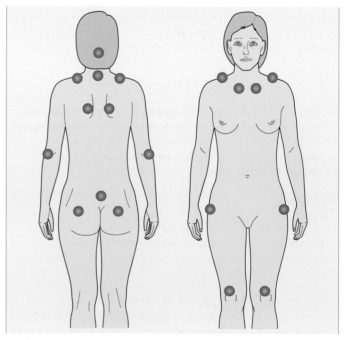

Distribution of hyperalgesic tender spots

diffuse musculoskeletal pain or tenderness of no identified cause. Pain is a constant feature that can be exacerbated by emotional and physical stressors. Patients are always tired and find it difficult to perform everyday activities. Other symptoms, including headaches and irritable bowel syndrome, will have resulted in consultations with other hospital specialists.

Cause

The cause of fibromyalgia continues to be debated and whether it is a distinct clinical entity lacks consensus. It is unlikely to be related to a single factor. A marked sex difference is seen, with more women than men diagnosed with the syndrome: ratios of 7:1 are reported. Triggers include trauma and emotional distress. It has been postulated that a previous traumatic experience may modulate the expression and perpetuation of pain in susceptible individuals. A 1994 review paper analysing British publications identified that 49% of publications favoured a non-organic cause, with 31% focusing on an organic cause. In total, 80% of the popular press favoured an organic explanation. The similarities between fibromyalgia and chronic fatigue syndrome have been noted, and whether the syndromes are identical expressions of the same process is under debate.

Management

The absence of an obvious source of ongoing nociception or inflammation makes the application of a medical model inappropriate, and the clinical significance of research studies is often difficult to interpret. No standardised effective treatments exist for the symptoms of fibromyalgia. Management focuses on returning control to the individual through the development of coping strategies. This involves the use of a biopsychosocial approach to address all dimensions of the pain experience. A Cochrane review of multidisciplinary rehabilitation in fibromyalgia concluded that behavioural treatments and stress management are important components.

In primary care, risk factors for the development of fibromyalgia can be identified at an early stage, with appropriate strategies implemented, including lifestyle advice on, for example, exercise and stress management skills. Studies suggest a more favourable outcome for patients maintained in a community setting. Only patients with increasing functional impairment will need a specific multidisciplinary integrated programme, which is often offered within secondary care.

Management strategies

Descriptive and experimental studies support a multimodal programme of management including physical, psychological, and educational components delivered in a multidisciplinary setting. Components of such programmes include education, pacing of activities, exercise, and relaxation.

Education

The patient will need guidance, support, and motivation from a health professional to adopt a different perspective towards their symptoms and begin the active process of self-management. This process involves learning problem solving techniques and behavioural skills. Often the patient will have stopped functioning, have become trapped by their pain, and be displaying illness behaviour. It is important that the relation between psychosocial factors and pain perception is discussed, as this can often be influenced by the patient's own behaviour and attitude towards the problem.

Theories about cause of fibromyalgia

- Neuroendocrine disturbance
    Neurohormonal dysfunctions
    Abnormal pain processing
    Autonomic nervous system dysfunction
- Sleep physiology
    Electroencephelographic evidence of reduced non-rapid eye movement sleep
- Muscle pathology
    Changes in regulation of intramuscular microcirculation
    Decrease in energy rich phosphates
- Allergy, infection, toxicity, and nutritional deficiency
- Psychosomatic
- Trauma
    Whiplash
- Neurotransmitter regulation

Risk factors for fibromyalgia

- Family history
- Sleep disturbance
- Work-related pain
- Emotional distress
- Stress

Coping strategies

- Exercise
- Pacing
- Diversional therapy
- Goal setting
- Relaxation
- Cognitive restructuring

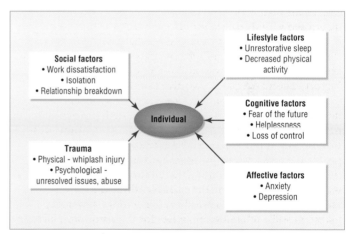

Possible mechanism for perpetuation of musculoskeletal distress

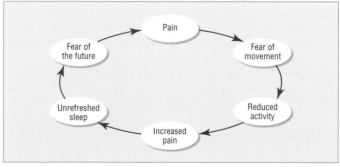

Pain cycle

Pacing of activities

Pacing involves breaking down everyday activities into achievable components through the planning and pacing of activities. It removes the "all or nothing mentality" patients use to reduce pain and fatigue. Patients are encouraged to engage in a balanced programme of purposeful activity that is achievable and realistic. This reinforces a sense of accomplishment, and the patient will be able to increase their activity in a structured way and regain control of the situation.

Exercise

The aim of graded exercise (that is gradually increasing activity over time) is to improve the patient's general physical fitness and resistance to small traumas, while increasing their strength, stamina, and flexibility. This ultimately leads to higher levels of general activity. Several sessions of supervised exercise may be needed at first to encourage motivation and provide feedback.

Relaxation

Many studies advocate relaxation in the management of fibromyalgia. It gives patients a strategy to reduce muscle tension and stress, improve sleep, cope with panic attacks (through controlled breathing), and reduce awareness of pain.

Complementary and alternative medicine

Up to 91% of patients with fibromyalgia use complementary and alternative therapies; this compares with 63% of patients with rheumatological disorders. Cognitive behavioural therapy reduces feelings of anxiety and depression. Randomised controlled trials showed that acupuncture can reduce objective and subjective measures of pain in some patients, but in others, it exacerbates symptoms. No strong evidence supports the use of manipulative techniques such as chiropractic and massage.

Drug management

Pharmacological treatments are not particularly successful. Randomised controlled trials showed that subtherapeutic doses of tricyclic antidepressants (for example, amitriptyline) and combinations (for example, amitriptyline plus fluoxetine) improve pain, fatigue, and quality of sleep, but improvements are not maintained in the long term. Antidepressants are often tolerated poorly and patients stop using them. If they are used, the doctor should explain the aim of the intervention: to help sleep and pain perception rather than to treat depression. A trial of a tricyclic for 3-4 months is advocated; the patient should start with small doses of 10 mg, with the possibility of increasing gradually to 50 mg at night in some cases. The decision to increase the dose will be based on efficacy and side effects. Even with low doses, side effects—are common. Patients with fibromyalgia use analgesics on a fairly regular basis, despite their lack of efficacy. They may start this habit to add credibility to the pain being experienced. Simple analgesics, such as paracetamol, may be prescribed, but stronger narcotics should be avoided.

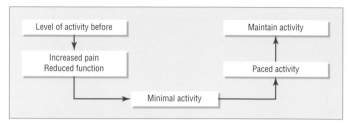

Pacing activities

Predictors of chronic illness behaviour
- Psychological distress
- Poor self reported health
- Low levels of physical activity
- Length of pain duration

Psychosocial influences on pain
- Anxiety
- Depression
- Low self esteem
- Feelings of helplessness
- Loss of control

Side effects of antidepressants
- Dry mouth
- Constipation
- Fluid retention
- Weight gain

Conclusion

Fibromyalgia syndrome is a challenge to both the patient and doctor. Effective self-management of symptoms that results in physical, psychological, and social functioning is the goal of management. In terms of management strategies, evidence suggests the need for an integrated programme of care that uses the skills of a multidisciplinary team to develop effective coping strategies. Further systematic evaluation of the effectiveness of non-pharmacological interventions is needed.

The figure showing the distribution of hyperalgesic tender spots is adapted from a figure in a patient booklet published by the Arthritis Research Campaign on Fibromyalgia.

Further reading

- McClean G, Wessely S. Professional and popular view of CFS. *BMJ* 1994;308:776-7
- American College of Rheumatology. Criteria for the classification of fibromyalgia. *Arthritis Rheum* 1990;33:160-72
- Wigers SH, Stiles TC, Vogel PA. Effects of aerobic exercise versus stress management in fibromyalgia. A 4.5 year prospective study. *Scand J Rheumatol* 1996;25:77-86
- Nicassio PM, Radojevic V, Weisman MH, Schuman C, Kim J, Schoenfeld-Smith K, et al. A comparison of behavioural and education interventions for fibromyalgia. *J Rheumatol* 1997;24:2000-7
- Chaitow L. *Fibromyalgia syndrome: a practitioner's guide to treatment.* Edinburgh: Churchill Livingstone, 2000.
- Wolfe F, Ross K, Anderson J, Russell IJ, Herbert L. The prevalence and characteristics of fibromyalgia in the general population. *Arthritis Rheum* 1995;38:19-28
- Granges G, Zilko P, Littlejohn GO. Fibromyalgia syndrome assessment of the severity of the condition and two years after diagnosis. *J Rheumatol* 1994;21:523-9
- Goldenberg DL. A randomised double-blind cross over trial of fluoxetine and amitriptyline in the treatment of fibromyalgia. *Arthritis Rheum* 1996;39:1852-9
- Arnold LM, Keck PE, Welge JA. Antidepressant treatment of fibromyalgia. A meta analysis and review. *Psychosomatics* 2000;41:104-13
- Sim J, Adams N. Physical and other non-pharmacological interventions for Fibromyalgia. *Bailliére's Best Pract Res Clin Rheumatol* 1999;13:507-23

8 Osteoarthritis

Nicholas Raj, Adrian Jones

Osteoarthritis is probably a final common pathway that results from a heterogeneous group of overlapping conditions. It is the most common condition to affect synovial joints, the most important cause of locomotor disability, and a major challenge for healthcare providers. Osteoarthritis was considered to be a degenerative disease that was an inevitable consequence of ageing and trauma, but it is viewed now as a metabolically dynamic, essentially reparative process that is increasingly amenable to treatment. The pathological changes are produced by local cytokines and proteases, so although osteoarthritis is probably driven mechanically, it is mediated biochemically.

No definition of osteoarthritis is accepted generally, but most would agree that pathologically it is a condition of synovial joints characterised by focal cartilage loss and an accompanying reparative bone response. In practice, the definition is less straightforward. Current diagnosis hinges on detection of structural changes clinically or in radiographs. For many doctors, the plain radiograph remains the best means of assessment, with evidence of cartilage loss (joint space narrowing) and bone response (presence of osteophytes and sclerosis) being the main criteria. This definition, however, excludes joints with early minimal change, ignores tissues other than cartilage and bone, and does not consider biological consequences (symptoms and disability). Often discordance between structural change and clinical outcome is considerable; patients with apparent structural catastrophe may have few or no symptoms, and often too much importance is given to radiographic changes.

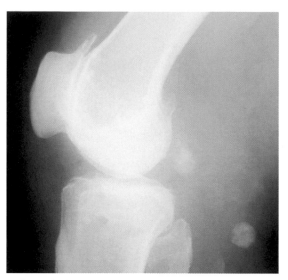

Radiograph of joint affected by osteoarthritis

A better understanding of the causes of symptoms and disability of osteoarthritis is still a key challenge

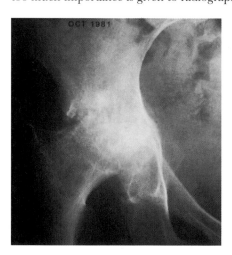 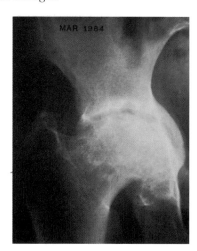

Example of healing osteoarthritis at the hip joint. Note reappearance of a wider joint space, implying growth of new articular cartilage. This is likely to be fibro-cartilage, rather than hyaline cartilage

Process of osteoarthritis

Observations about osteoarthritis have led to the suggestion that it is an aspect of the inherent repair process of synovial joints. In most cases, this slow but metabolically active process keeps pace with various triggering insults and is non-progressive, but sometimes it fails to compensate and this results in joint failure and associated symptoms and disability. This interpretation partly explains the heterogeneity of osteoarthritis: various extrinsic and intrinsic insults cause different patterns of arthritis and multiple constitutional and environmental factors modify response and outcome.

Observations about osteoarthritis

- Present throughout evolution and ubiquitous in humans and other vertebrates
- Not simply attrition of joint structures but a metabolically active condition that shows variable balance between anabolic and catabolic processes—at different stages, activity is increased in all joint tissues (cartilage, bone, synovium, capsule, and muscle)
- Common but usually asymptomatic
- Occasionally, radiographs show "healing" of osteoarthritic joints

Osteoarthritis targets specific joints—possibly those that have undergone recent evolutionary changes in function (particularly relating to bipedal locomotion and precision grip) but have not yet adapted adequately.

Risk factors

Age
Although not an inevitable consequence of ageing, osteoarthritis is strongly related to age. This may represent the cumulative effect of insults to the joint, possibly aggravated by decline in neuromuscular function, or senescence of homoeostatic repair mechanisms. The consequence is a considerable medical burden that will increase as the number of elderly people in the British population increases.

Sex
The female preponderance for severe radiographic grades of osteoarthritis overall, osteoarthritis of the hand and knee radiographically, and symptoms is pronounced.

Ethnic groups
Osteoarthritis of the hip is less common in black and Asian populations than in white populations, and polyarticular osteoarthritis of the hand is rare in black Africans and Malaysians. This difference seems to reflect genetic rather than cultural differences.

Individual risk factors
Two main categories of such risk factors exist:

- generalised factors (for example, obesity, genetic factors, and female sex)
- localised factors that result in abnormal mechanical loading at specific sites (such as meniscectomy and instability).

Trauma is a predisposing factor that may localise the affected site in those likely to develop osteoarthritis. For example, trauma in college years is related to an increase in the prevalence of osteoarthritis in the sixtieth decade; this suggests that measures to reduce trauma, especially that secondary to sporting activity, may be important in reducing future disease.

Various professions have been linked with an increased incidence of osteoarthritis: osteoarthritis of the hip and farming has the strongest association, and it is now considered as an industrial disease. Certain sports played at a professional level may increase the risk of osteoarthritis even when trauma has been taken into consideration, for example, football and osteoarthritis of the knee. That moderate sports activity that does not result in joint injury is unlikely to be a significant risk factor must be stressed, however; the benefits of aerobic exercise probably outweigh any detrimental effects of repetitive joint loading.

The genetics of osteoarthritis is unknown, but a strong inherited component to osteoarthritis of the hand, knee, and hip has been demonstrated, especially for osteoarthritis that involves multiple joints. That these conditions are not monogenic is clear, and osteoarthritis is likely to be the result of a polygenic predisposition to the development of clinical disease. Some factors (such as obesity, muscle function, and occupation) may be modified and thus offer scope for primary, secondary, and tertiary prevention.

Types of osteoarthritis

Despite attempts to subdivide osteoarthritis according to various criteria, no sharp divisions exist in the spectrum of

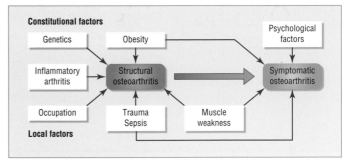

Pathogenesis of osteoarthritis

Prevalence of osteoarthritis

- Osteoarthritis is uncommon (and multiple joint osteoarthritis is rare) in people <45 years
- Prevalence of osteoarthritis increases up to age 65, when at least half of people have radiographic evidence of osteoarthritis in at least one joint group
- Prevalence of symptomatic osteoarthritis also increases with age, but data for this association are less clear (for example, the knee is affected in about 15% of people >55 years)
- Increases in prevalence (symptomatic and asymptomatic osteoarthritis) over the age of 65 are less clear

Putative risk factors for the development and progression of hip and knee osteoarthritis

Stage of disease	Hip	Knee
Development	• Previous disease or trauma (such as Perthes' disease or slipped femoral epiphysis) • Avascular necrosis	• Previous trauma (such as meniscectomy) • Medial femoral necrosis • Sex (female) • Non-gonococcal septic arthritis
Progression	• Non-gonococcal septic arthritis • Occupation (farming) • Superior pole pattern • Chondrocalcinosis (knee)	• Occupational knee bending and lifting • Obesity • Valgus and varus alignment • Chondrocalcinosis • Use of non-steroidal anti-inflammatory drugs

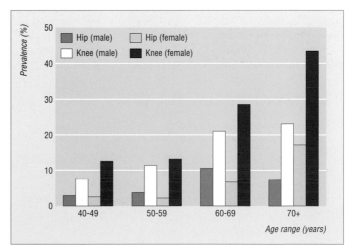

Prevalence of radiographic evidence of osteoarthritis

osteoarthritis. People may display different features at different sites and evolve from one "subset" to another. Nevertheless certain distinctions may be useful.

Nodal generalised osteoarthritis (menopausal osteoarthritis)

This common condition clusters in families. Its outcome, particularly with respect to hand symptoms and function, is generally good. A strong inherited pattern is seen, and work is under way to identify genetic associations.

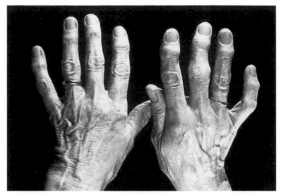

Nodal generalised osteoarthritis

Characteristics of nodal generalised osteoarthritis

- Multiple Heberden's nodes (distal interphalangeal joints)
- Bouchard's nodes (proximal interphalangeal joints)
- Symptoms start around time of menopause
- Polyarticular osteoarthritis of interphalangeal joints
- Later development of osteoarthritis of knee, hip, and apophyseal joint

---

Crystal associated osteoarthritis

Calcium crystals, notably calcium pyrophosphate dihydrate and apatite, may deposit in cartilage as an isolated phenomenon, but they also occur often in osteoarthritic joints. In this context, they probably arise through physicochemical changes that accompany the osteoarthritis process. Although these crystals may sometimes initiate inflammation (such as in acute pseudogout), they usually have no direct deleterious effects.

Osteoarthritis with deposition of calcium pyrophosphate dihydrate (pyrophosphate arthropathy) occurs predominantly in elderly women, principally affects the knee, and is associated with inflammation and widespread and pronounced radiographic (usually hypertrophic) changes.

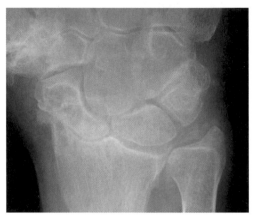

Radiograph of wrist showing chondrocalcinosis and arthropathy

Apatite associated destructive arthritis

Although modest amounts of apatite are present in most osteoarthritic joints, large amounts occur in apatite associated destructive arthritis. This is almost totally confined to the hips, shoulders (Milwaukee shoulder), and knees of elderly women, and it has a poor outcome. Rapid painful progression with large cool effusions, progressive instability, and atrophic radiographic changes are seen typically. The differential diagnosis includes Charcot arthropathy, sepsis, and avascular necrosis.

Osteoarthritis of premature onset

Development of single joint osteoarthritis after severe trauma or alteration in joint biomechanics (for example, after meniscectomy or because of developmental abnormality) is not uncommon. Premature onset (in people <50 years) in several joints, however, should prompt consideration of predisposing metabolic, hormonal, or other causes. Conditions for which osteoarthritis of premature onset can be the presenting feature are rare. Some are amenable to correction (although existing osteoarthritis is usually unaffected).

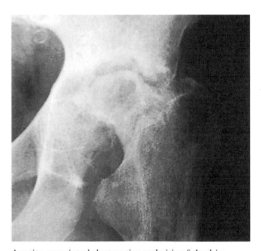

Apatite associated destructive arthritis of the hip

Clinical features

The main clinical features of osteoarthritis are symptoms, functional impairment, and signs. Considerable discordance can exist between these three. Pain may arise from several sites in and around an osteoarthritic joint. Suggested mechanisms include increased capsular and intraosseous pressure, subchondral microfracture, and enthesopathy or bursitis secondary to muscle weakness and structural alteration. Severity of pain and functional impairment are greatly influenced by personality, anxiety, depression, daily activity, muscle strength, and abnormal proprioception.

Conditions for which osteoarthritis of premature onset is a presenting feature

- Haemochromatosis
- Ochronosis
- Acromegaly
- Spondyloepiphyseal dysplasia, epiphyseal dysplasia, and hereditary type II collagen defects
- Thiemann's disease
- Endemic osteoarthritis (normally rare but common in endemic areas)

Crepitus, bony enlargement, deformity, instability, and restricted movement may occur together and predominantly reflect structural changes. Varying degrees of synovitis (warmth, effusion, and synovial thickening) may be superimposed, and muscle weakness or wasting is usual. Periarticular sources of pain are present, often at the knee and hip.

Assessment

Assessment aims to establish the source of symptoms in each patient. Determination of the presence of osteoarthritis is not often a problem—the usual question is whether osteoarthritis is relevant to the patient's complaints. The high prevalence of osteoarthritis in the general population means that co-morbid conditions often exist. These include soft tissue lesions (enthesopathy and bursitis), fibromyalgia, gout, inflammatory arthritis, and sepsis, and need attention in their own right. Only an adequate history and examination can determine how much structural and inflammatory change is present and how much this contributes to a patient's problems.

Treatment

The aims of treatment are patient education, pain relief, optimisation of function, and minimisation of progression.

Patient education and psychological factors
The myth that osteoarthritis is a progressive wearing out of joints due to old age still persists; this invariably leads to inappropriate reductions in activity. A major contribution to managing osteoarthritis has been the finding that a patient's psychological status (anxiety, depression, and social support) is an important determinant of symptomatic and functional outcome. Good evidence supports the use of educational programmes to help patients understand and develop self-management strategies.

Biomechanical factors
Weight reduction is desirable in obese patients and may reduce progression of knee osteoarthritis. Loss of muscle strength is associated with disability. Strength and aerobic fitness, which are beneficial to osteoarthritic joints and personal well being, can be increased in all age groups. Insoles to counteract knee varus deformity, patello-femoral strapping, walking sticks, and cushioned shoes (trainers) can redistribute stress and reduce impact loading.

Pain control
Pain is the main reason patients seek help. The current high use of non-steroidal anti-inflammatory drugs for osteoarthritis is probably inappropriate. Regular doses of analgesics such as paracetamol are usually enough for most patients. Symptoms of osteoarthritis often are episodic, and if non-steroidal anti-inflammatory drugs are used the need for them should be re-evaluated regularly, especially in elderly patients who are at risk of side effects. Non-steroidal anti-inflammatory drugs more specific for cyclooxygenase-2 are alternatives for patients at higher risk of gastrointestinal side effects. No convincing evidence yet shows that non-steroidal anti-inflammatory drugs affect progression of osteoarthritis in humans, but hastening of progression (especially by indomethacin) has been suggested. Topical non-steroidal anti-inflammatory drugs have similar efficacy to oral preparations in patients with osteoarthritis, but as they have fewer side effects, they should be used more often, particularly for patients with a few symptomatic and readily

---

Assessment of patients with osteoarthritis

Nature of pain
- Mechanical—related to use
- Inflammatory—stiffness and pain aggravated by rest
- Nocturnal—suggests interosseous hypertension
- Sudden deterioration—consider sepsis, avascular necrosis, fracture, or crystal synovitis

Clinical examination
- Periarticular or articular source of pain?
- Generalised pain—consider fibromyalgia (test tender sites)
- Presence of deformity?
- Evidence of muscle wasting?
- Local inflammation or effusion?
- Generalised or localised osteoarthritis?

Joint locking
- Orthopaedic referral probably appropriate

Weight
- Potentially modifiable risk factor

Sleep disturbance
- May be associated with fibromyalgia and depression

Co-morbid disease
- Modifies risk of treatment with non-steroidal anti-inflammatory drugs and of surgery
- May be evidence of disease associated with premature osteoarthritis (for example, haemochromatosis)

Aims of treatment
- Patient education
- Pain relief
- Optimisation of function
- Minimisation of progression

All people involved in the management of patients should give consistent advice and emphasise that the outlook for these conditions is considerably better than expected

---

Changes in lifestyle for patients with osteoarthritis

General measures
- Maintain optimal weight
- Encourage activity and regular general exercise
- Maintain positive approach

Specific measures
- Strengthening of local muscles
- Use of appropriate footwear and walking aids
- Pay attention to specific problems caused by disability (such as shopping, housework, and job)

accessible joints. Substantial doubt remains, however, about their superiority over simple rubefacients. Topical capsaicin may alleviate pain in osteoarthritis with few side effects.

Several other symptomatic treatments (some with claimed chondroprotective action) are available in some countries or are under investigation. Considerable interest is given to pharmacological manipulation of osteoarthritis (and exciting experimental data), but the precise role of such drugs in treatment is not yet defined. Glucosamine, which is available as a health food, is the best characterised of these. Trials of pharmacological grade glucosamine in Italy and the United States suggest symptomatic benefit and at least one American study noted a possible slowing of disease progression.

Disease modifying drugs
The use of intra-articular corticosteroid injections for uncomplicated osteoarthritis is controversial and generally not recommended. They have a place, however, in the treatment of patients with acute crystal associated synovitis or those who are unfit for or awaiting surgery. Hyaluronic acid preparations have been shown to have disease-modifying effects only in vitro and so at present have a similar role to intra-articular steroids, with a longer duration of action (six months).

Surgery
The success of prosthetic joint replacements has greatly advanced management of end stage hip and knee osteoarthritis. Surgery is also used increasingly now at the shoulder, elbow, and thumb base. Although issues of funding, waiting times, choice of prosthesis, and revision have to be faced, that such surgery can transform patients' lives is not in doubt. Other surgical approaches (arthroscopic lavage, osteotomy, and arthrodesis) may also be useful. Arthroscopy has the benefit of direct visualisation of the cartilage and associated structures facilitating surgical correction of meniscal or ligamentous injury, and the symptomatic improvement from joint lavage can be relatively longstanding. The criteria for surgery are not definite, but they probably should include uncontrolled pain (particularly nocturnal pain) and severe impairment of function. Age, in itself, is not a contraindication.

Drug treatments for osteoarthritis

- Adequate doses of simple analgesics (for example, acetaminophen)
- Topical preparations such as non-steroidal anti-inflammatory drugs, rubefacients, and capsaicin
- Non-steroidal anti-inflammatory drugs
  Only for patients with symptoms not controlled by other means or during acute exacerbations
  Use the lowest dose that controls symptoms
  Regularly review continued use
  Use cyclooxygenase-2 selective agents (currently rofecoxib, celecoxib, meloxicam, and etodolac) in patients at risk of gastrointestinal toxicity or who need long-term therapy
- Glucosamine
  Possibly has slow onset but sustained symptomatic benefit
  Available in United Kingdom as a health food
- Intra-articular corticosteroid injections
  Consider for patients unfit for surgery or for acute flares
- Intra-articular hyaluronic acid injections
  Expensive option but consider for those unfit for surgery

Surgical treatments for osteoarthritis

- History of joint locking
  Consider arthroscopy for removal of loose body
- Persistent synovitis
  Consider arthroscopic washout
- Joint replacement is highly effective for hip and knee
  Consider early referral for opinion
- Joint surgery also has a role at the thumb base, shoulder, and elbow

---

Further reading

- Altman, RD. Status of hyaluronan supplementation therapy in osteoarthritis. *Curr Rheumatol Rep* 2003;5:7-14
- American College of Rheumatology Subcommittee on Osteoarthritis Guidelines. Recommendations for the medical management of osteoarthritis of the hip and knee. 2000 Update. *Arthritis Rheum* 2000;43:1905-15
- Cooper C. Occupational activity and the risk of the osteoarthritis. *J Rheumatol* 1995;22:10-12
- Hurley MV. Quadriceps weakness in osteoarthritis. *Curr Op Rheumatol* 1998;10:246-50
- Klippel JH, Dieppe PA, eds. Osteoarthritis and related disorders in rheumatology. In *Rheumatology*. 2nd ed. London: Mosby, 1998:4.1-14.1
- McAlindon TE, LaValley MP, Gulin JP, Felson DT. Glucosamine and chondroitin for treatment of osteoarthritis: a systematic quality assessment and meta-analysis. *JAMA* 2000;283:1469-75
- Towheed TE, Anastassiades TP, Shea B, Houpt J, Welch V. Hochberg MC. Glucosamine therapy for treating osteoarthritis. *Cochrane Database of Systematic Reviews*, 2001
- Zhang WY, Po ALW. The effectiveness of topically applied capsaicin. *Eur J Clin Pharmacol* 1994;46:517-22

9 Gout and hyperuricaemia

Michael L Snaith, Adewale O Adebajo

The term "gout" is meant to include an acute attack, the propensity for repeated episodes, and also chronic gouty arthritis. The cause is inflammation induced by microcrystalline uric acid in the form of monosodium urate monohydrate in joints and soft tissues. A usual but not essential prerequisite for the condition is a raised plasma level of urate, which is derived from endogenous and dietary nucleoproteins. Patients with gout are also liable to develop various aspects of atherosclerosis. This chapter covers gouty inflammation and its treatment, the risks of hyperuricaemia and its management, and the non-gouty implications of circulating urate.

Considerations in patients with gout and hyperuricaemia
- Episodic acute inflammatory gouty arthritis
- Chronic inflammatory gouty arthritis
- Accumulated deposits of urate as tophi
- Damage to joints, soft tissues, and kidneys
- Renal and bladder stones
- Blood urate and its implications
- Associations with atherosclerosis and insulin resistance
- Treatment of gout and management of hyperuricaemia

Acute gouty arthritis

Acute gout is more painful than any form of arthritis—with the possible exception of septic arthritis. Typically, patients become aware of discomfort during the night and by the morning the affected joint is throbbing and inflamed. The great toe joint (first metatarsal phalangeal joint) is the site of the first attack of gout in ≥50% of cases and it also is affected at one time or another in 75% of cases of recurrent gout. Affected toe joints make it painful to walk or even wear shoes. Even with prompt treatment with effective anti-inflammatory drugs, symptoms may last 1-2 weeks or even longer. Untreated attacks can last several weeks.

The first attack of gout is often severe. The differential diagnosis is septic arthritis, as both conditions share the same characteristic acute, localised, rapidly increasing inflammation. In both diseases, polymorphonuclear effusion, which reacts to showering of urate crystals, is predominant. Sepsis must be excluded by negative microscopy for organisms and cultures to identify microorganisms and their sensitivity to antibiotics. The absolute diagnosis of gout needs polarising microscopy, which allows accurate and rapid confirmation of the presence of urate crystals in fluid or tissue. Urate crystals can also be detected with a conventional microscope by phase contrast or with a makeshift polariser and adhesive tape. Polarising light also allows urate gout and pseudogout, which is caused by crystals of pyrophosphate (see Chapter 8), to be discriminated. Both types of crystals coexist in perhaps 10% of synovial effusions.

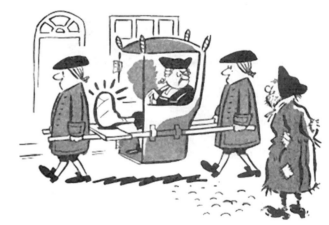

It affects more rich than poor

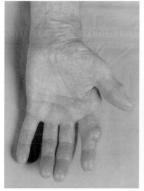
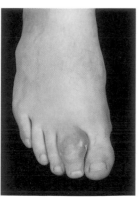

Chronic gouty arthritis

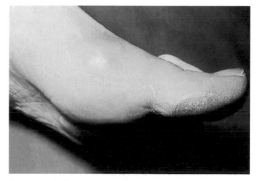

Acute gouty foot

Chronic, tophaceous, and polyarticular gout

Acute gout is usually but not exclusively monoarticular. Chronic, polyarticular gout is a common cause of inflammatory arthritis in older men, but it also should be considered in older women, especially those on diuretics. No diagnostic pattern exists, although a predilection for lower joint involvement is noted. An indicator for a diagnosis of chronic gouty arthritis is a history of evolution from acute episodic gout to chronicity or polyarticular involvement, but this is not predictably obtained. Tophi should be sought and are particularly common in older women with secondary, diuretic-induced gout, in whom they may develop with no persuasive history of acute gout. X ray examination is usually helpful, and diagnostic features may be seen in any suspicious joint. Erythrocyte sedimentation rates and levels of C reactive protein are variable.

> **Rheumatoid factor tests are essentially negative in gout, but beware of biological false positives in older patients and those with a family history of rheumatoid arthritis. Rheumatoid arthritis and gout can coexist**

Gout—then and now

The history of gout is a little romanticised by its socioeconomic connotations, but the typical patient has changed from the stereotypical view of the 17th-19th centuries and patients fall into one of three groups. Rare but individually important metabolic conditions may involve gout. The prevalence of gout is 5-10 per 1000 adults in the population in the United Kingdom. Men account for most young patients, but the number of women increases proportionally with age.

Changing face of the patient with gout

17th-19th centuries	20th-21st centuries
• Middle-aged to elderly rich, influential, obese, irascible male who overindulged in food and alcohol	• Young, otherwise well men perhaps with a family history of gout • Middle-aged somewhat obese men with hypertension and cardiovascular disease • Older men or women with gout secondary to diuretic use

Hyperuricaemia

Hyperuricaemia is defined not by the usual population mean plus two standard deviations, but by the solubility of urate in plasma or serum. Urate is a weak acid that dissociates in solution, but in plasma, urate theoretically exceeds its solubility product above about 6.5 mg/100 ml (368 μmol/l) because of the high level of sodium. Levels >420 μmol/l (7.0 mg/100 ml) in men and 340 μmol/l (5.7 mg/100 ml) in women are considered as being hyperuricaemic. In males, blood urate rises at puberty to adult levels, whereas in females, only a drift upwards is seen until the menopause, when the level rises to closer to that seen in men.

Some factors that influence blood levels of urate

- Body weight
- Body mass index
- Diet (purines, lipids, alcohol)
- Medication (diuretics, antituberculosis drugs)
- Hypertension
- Renal function
- Ketosis

Hyperuricaemia and gout worldwide

Caution should be exercised in the interpretation of point prevalences of gout in different populations, as they have been surveyed with various study designs, criteria, and methods. Data show striking differences, however, in the prevalence rates of gout and hyperuricaemia in various populations.

Gout was not recorded in Polynesians of the South Pacific Islands and New Zealand before 1914. Now, these populations have some of the highest rates of gout and hyperuricaemia. Maoris are predisposed to hyperuricaemia: one in three men aged >40 years is affected and the overall frequency of gout in men is about 10%—more than eight times the frequency in age matched counterparts in Europe and North America or in New Zealanders of European stock. Elsewhere in the Pacific, on the island of Nauru, 7% of men have gout and 64% of men and 60% of women aged >20 years have hyperuricaemia—the highest prevalences reported for any population.

Most authors suggest that these high prevalences are related to changes from the traditional island style of living towards westernisation. This point was dramatically reinforced in a study of the incidence in Tokelauans that lasted 14 years. From

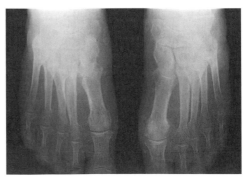

X ray radiograph of gouty joint showing bony erosion

a baseline of around 20:1000, the prevalence of gout rose to 51:1000 in migrated Tokelauan males compared with a fall to 15:1000 in non-migrated males over the same period. The relative risk of gout was nine times higher in the migrant Tokelauans, which placed them in the same risk class as the New Zealand Maoris. Studies of age specific incidence showed that gout occurs at an early age in migrant men. The prevalence and incidence changes in clinical gout are matched by significantly higher levels of uric acid in the serum of migrants than in non-migrants. Perhaps indigenous Polynesians of the Pacific Basin form one large potentially gouty group.

The Malayo Polynesians of Java also have high rates of gout and hyperuricaemia, despite the lack of alcohol consumption and very low meat consumption. These observations imply that other, probably genetic, factors operate in these indigenous populations. The clearance rate of urate in Maori men is lower in patients with gout, which suggests that susceptibility to hyperuricaemia has a renal mechanism. Even in Maoris with normal levels of uric acid in serum, renal clearance is similar to values obtained in British males with gout. This might explain the fundamental tendency of Polynesians to hyperuricaemia.

In Africa, sporadic case reports before 1980 suggested gout was a rare disease, although lack of awareness and misdiagnosis are potential explanations. Socioeconomic considerations do not seem to be relevant among Africans. In sub-Saharan Africa in general and South Africa in particular, gout is associated with alcohol consumption across the entire social and economic strata. An overwhelming predominance of gout in men is also seen in Africa, where gout is 6-19 times more common in men than women depending on the African country studied. A high prevalence of urate stones is found in Israel.

In Malaysia, the three largest ethnic groups are Malays, Chinese, and Tamils. All have higher mean levels of uric acid in serum than most Caucasian populations. In contrast, black Africans, Japanese, and Native Americans generally have lower levels than Caucasian populations. Acculturation may have led to higher levels of uric acid in serum in Filipinos, Malayo mongoloids, Tokelauans, Polynesians, and Chinese mongoloids.

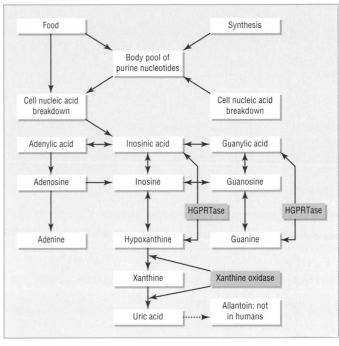

Metabolic pathway of uric acid. Uric acid is not a normal human dietary constituent. The body pool is derived from dietary purines and breakdown of endogenous nucleic acids. HGPRTase=hypoxanthine guanine phosphoribosyl transferase

Origin and elimination of urate

Humans and some primates lack uricase, which in other species degrades urate to allantoin. Birds and reptiles excrete urate as their major nitrogen elimination product. Humans are in a state of near urate intolerance and may suffer from this in a number of ways. Nucleoproteins degrade to pyrimidines, oxipurines (xanthine and hypoxanthine), and then to uric acid via xanthine oxidase, the target for allopurinol. Sources of purine are exogenous intake and endogenous catabolism. Adult males produce around 1.2 g of purine daily, of which 200-600 mg is urinary. Lower gut bacteria degrade most intestinal purine, so gut reabsorption is usually clinically unimportant. The total product of purine may rise if the breakdown of nucleoprotein exceeds physiological salvage pathways. This is particularly likely when rapid reductions of circulating or solid tumour mass occurs during radiotherapy or chemotherapy for haematological malignancies. This "secondary" gout can be prevented by prophylactic allopurinol.

Renal clearance of urate is normally total at the glomerulus. Proximal tubular reabsorption is followed by distal re-excretion, so urinary levels depend upon the resultant flux and are influenced by urine flow, pH, and competition for tubular exchange. Other dissociated weak acids, such as lactate, reduce urate tubular excretion and so cause a rise in plasma urate.

Manifestations of urate intolerance

- Gouty arthritis
- Renal stones
- Cardiovascular disorders
- Insulin resistance syndromes

Hyperuricaemia is not diagnostic for gout

Gout can occur without hyperuricaemia

Urinary levels of urate are normal in 80% of patients with hyperuricaemia and gout, which means they have a reduced rate of urate clearance. This raises the question as to whether primary gout is caused by a primary renal abnormality, a primary abnormality of purine metabolism, or a secondary tubular defect. The probable answer is that some or all may coexist in different patients.

Hyperuricaemia, hyperuricosuria, and renal stones

Around 20% of patients overexcrete urate (more than 600 mg/4000 μmol in 24 hours) and they are especially prone to urate stones. Urate solubility is considerably influenced by pH, and patients with gout tend to excrete acid urine: another argument for a renal defect as a cause in gout. Concentrated acidic urine is predictive of urate stones, as is seen in dehydrated patients and those with ileostomies.

Primary and secondary gout and inherited metabolic disorders that present with gout

The terms primary and secondary may be somewhat confusing. Gout in childhood may be a manifestation of one of the several rare metabolic disorders of purine metabolism and should be investigated in detail. Adults with new onset gout may be heterozygous for one of these conditions but investigations should be restricted to those with indicative family histories.

Risks of hyperuricaemia

Acute gout is unlikely to occur below a level of urate in blood of about 300 μmol/l (5.0 mg/100 ml), but no absolute level is diagnostic of gout. The likelihood of gout being present rises to near-inevitability above around 550 μmol/l, but that does not dictate when the first attack will occur. About 10% of acute attacks occur with normal urate levels, especially soon after the introduction of urate lowering drugs (see below). The argument for routine screening is weak, and a diagnosis of gout should not hinge on the level of urate in the blood.

Treatment

Acute gout
Non-steroidal anti-inflammatory drugs are the first line choice for the treatment of acute gout. The initial dose needed is usually at least twice the normal maintenance dose, but attention must be paid to risk factors such as dyspepsia or fluid retention, and the dose should be tapered down as the pain diminishes. Colchicine is effective but often not tolerated at its full dose. Oral or parenteral steroids also are effective, but septic arthritis must be excluded positively, especially before intra-articular steroid is administered. Injection of intra-articular steroid is difficult and painful in smaller joints.

Repeated acute attacks and chronic gouty arthritis
Once the risks and benefits have been explained, a patient may opt for treatment of occasional attacks of acute gout rather than long-term maintenance with urate lowering drugs. Daily low dose colchicine is occasionally preferred. Long-term

A primary renal abnormality, a primary abnormality of purine metabolism, or a secondary tubular defect many coexist in patients. For example, lead poisoning causes a tubular defect, hyperuricaemia, and secondary gout. This "saturnine gout" occurs in people who drink the moonshine liquor brewed in many parts of the world, but best known in the southern states of the United States and in Australia. Lead poisoning may also have contributed to the development of gout in the 17th and 18th centuries because of lead contamination of wine and water in plumbing systems

Although only about 5% of renal stones are pure urate, raised levels of urate in the urine may coprecipitate calcium oxalate or phosphate stones

Risks of hyperuricaemia
- Episodic acute gout
- Episodic acute gout, leading to chronic gouty arthritis
- Urate stone formation in renal tract

Treatment of acute gouty arthritis
In order of preference:
1 Any non-steroidal anti-inflammatory drug at 2-3 times the maintenance dose for three days, then maintenance dose until resolution
2 Colchicine 0.5-1.0 mg orally every six hours for 24-48 hours, if tolerated
3 Intramuscular prednisolone acetate 125 mg immediately, or depot prednisolone 40-80 mg immediately
4 Oral prednisolone 30 mg daily, tapering to zero over 10 days

ingestion of non-steroidal anti-inflammatory drugs is more risky than urate reduction.

Why treat hyperuricaemia?

Hyperuricaemia is a marker of cardiovascular risk. This was thought to be because of an association with obesity and lifestyle; however, urate may associate with insulin resistance at the level of the renal tubule, which implies a metabolic cause. An attack of gout should also be regarded as an opportunity for reviewing the general health of the sufferer.

Diet and lifestyle

Diet has a definite place in the management of most patients with primary gout, both in diminishing the severity of acute gout and in reducing cardiovascular risk. A strict low intake of purine reduces plasma urate by about 20%. Although this can reduce the risk of gout usefully, it is difficult to sustain and may increase cardiovascular risk. Weight reduction to a body mass index $((weight\ (kg))/(height\ (m)^2))$ <25 is beneficial in general terms. After a diet with a relative increase in protein intake and no special emphasis on purine content, in which calories were restricted and saturated fats replaced by unsaturated fats, levels of urate and lipids in plasma and the number of attacks of gout were reduced.

Alcohol intake is relevant in terms of its contribution to obesity and purine intake and because of its metabolic effects. Many beers contain guanosine, which is converted into uric acid by gut bacteria. Alcohol taken without food is catabolised to lactate and other ketones that compete with urate for excretion by the renal tubule. Alcohol also decreases the conversion of allopurinol to the effective metabolite oxipurinol. Fortified wines may contain oxalates, which contribute to formation of stones. Coffee and tea are diuretics, so they also interfere with assays for urate.

Long-term pharmacological reduction of urate levels

Allopurinol is the market leader; however, hypersensitivity that produces rash and vasculitis can be troublesome, urate overproducers may be controlled inadequately, and xanthine stones remain a slight but definite risk. Uricosuric drugs thus still have a place. Benzbromarone has largely been overlooked in the United Kingdom. It is more potent than probenecid or sulphinpyrazone, and it may be used in patients with renal impairment and in conjunction with allopurinol. It inevitably increases the risk of stone formation, however, so a high fluid intake is important, and alkalinisation of urine is advisable. When a hypertensive patient with mild gout is treated, it is worth noting that the angiotensin II receptor antagonist losartan is mildly uricosuric, and this may offset the effects of thiazides. Another relevant observation is that fenofibrate is usefully uricosuric.

The gouty patient cartoon is reproduced with permission from the Arthritis Research Campaign.

Measures for long-term reduction of urate levels

Xanthine oxidase inhibition
- Allopurinol 100 mg/day, increasing to 200 mg/day up to a usual dose of 300 mg/day (may increase to 900 mg/day in divided doses)

Increase urate excretion with a uricosuric drug
- Probenecid 0.5-2.0 g/day
- Sulphinpyrazone 100-600 mg/day
- Benzbromarone 100 mg/day (named patient prescription in United Kingdom)

Note:
- Always suppress acute gout before starting urate reduction
- Risk that acute gout may be precipitated for <1 year, so always cover urate reduction with non-steroidal anti-inflammatory drug (maintenance dose) or colchicine (0.5-1.5 mg/day) for at least six months.

Associations of hyperuricaemia with or without hyperuricosuria

- Hypertension
- Hyperlipidaemia
- Coronary artery disease
- Peripheral vascular disease
- Cerebrovascular disease
- Syndrome X
- Insulin resistance

Dietary advice is important for most patients with gout, and may be sufficient for prevention of attacks in some

Alcohol is linked with gout and hyperuricaemia in several different ways

Pharmacological treatment of hyperuricaemia is indicated for most, but not all, patients with hyperuricaemia and gout. Alternatives to allopurinol are available, if required

---

Useful websites

- www.amg.gda.pl/~essppmm/ (accessed 18 November 2003)
  Website of European Society for the Study of Purine and Pyrimidine Metabolism in Man (ESSPPMM). It includes information on metabolic disorders and on diagnostic services in the European Union
- www.pumpa.co.uk
  Website of Purine Metabolic Patients Association, aimed at those with or relatives with rarer metabolic disorders
- www.ssiem.org.uk/ (accessed 18 November 2003)
  Website of Society for the Study of Inborn Errors of Metabolism
- www.ukgoutsociety.org
  Website of the UK Gout Society

Further reading

- Porter R, Rousseau GS. *Gout: the patrician malady.* New Haven: Yale University Press, 1998
- Wyngaarden JB, Kelley WN. *Gout and hyperuricaemia* Grune and Stratton: New York, 1976
- Grahame R, Simmonds HA, McBride MB, Marsh FP. How should we treat tophaceous gout in patients with allopurinol hypersensitivity? *Adv Exp Med Biol* 1998;431:19-23
- Facchini F, Chen Y-D, Hollenbeck CB, Reaven GM. Relationship between resistance to insulin-mediated glucose uptake, urinary uric acid clearance and plasma uric acid concentration. *JAMA* 1991;266:3008-11
- Yamashita S, Matsuzawa Y, Tokunaga K, Fujioka S, Tarui S. Studies on the impaired metabolism of uric acid in obese subjects: marked reduction of renal urate excretion and its improvement by a low-calorie diet. *Int J Obes* 1986;10:255-64
- Dessein PH, Shipton EA, Stanwix AE, Joffe BI, Ramokgadi J. Beneficial effects of weight loss associated with moderate calorie/carbohydrate restriction, and increased proportional intake of protein and unsaturated fat on serum urate and lipoprotein levels in gout: a pilot study. *Ann Rheum Dis* 2000;59:539-43
- Gutman AB, Yu T-F. Renal function in gout, with a commentary on the renal regulation of uretic excretion in the role of the kidney in the pathogenesis of gout. *Am J Med* 1957;23:600-22
- Grahame R, Simmonds HA, Carrey EA. *Gout at your fingertips.* London: Class Publishing Ltd, 2003

10 Osteoporosis

Nicola Peel, Richard Eastell

Osteoporotic fractures cause considerable morbidity and mortality. Recent estimates suggest that the cost of managing such fractures in the United Kingdom is over £1.7 billion a year.

Osteoporosis is a systemic skeletal disease characterised by low bone mass and micro-architectural deterioration that results in a high risk of fracture. Diagnosis is generally based on thresholds developed by the World Health Organization, in which a person's bone mineral density is compared with the mean (peak bone mass) for a young adult, as a standard deviation score (T score).

These thresholds were developed for measurements of bone mineral densities of the spine, hip, or forearm made with x ray based techniques in postmenopausal women. It is probably appropriate to use the same thresholds for bone mineral density measurements made in men and premenopausal women, but they should not be used for children or adolescents.

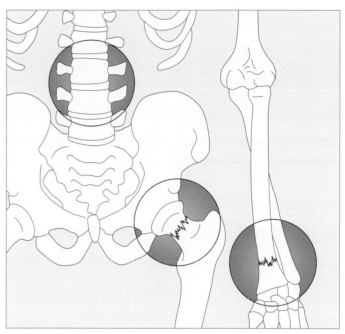

Typical sites of osteoporotic fracture

World Health Organization's diagnostic thresholds

Diagnosis	Bone mineral density T score (SD units)
Normal	> -1
Osteopenia	-1 to -2.5
Osteoporosis	< -2.5
Severe osteoporosis	< -2.5 plus one or more fragility fractures

Pathophysiology

The human skeleton is composed of approximately 20% trabecular bone and 80% cortical bone. Bone undergoes a continual process of resorption and formation in discrete bone remodelling units. Approximately 10% of the adult skeleton is remodelled per year. This turnover prevents fatigue damage and is important in maintaining calcium homeostasis. Irreversible bone loss results from an imbalance between the rates of resorption and formation. Trabecular bone is the more metabolically active, and osteoporotic fractures tend to occur at sites that contain more than 50% trabecular bone.

Bone loss leads to thinning, and often perforation, of the trabecular plates. Trabecular perforation occurs particularly in

Pattern of bone loss

- Peak bone mass is achieved by age 30 in the axial skeleton and earlier at appendicular sites
- After skeletal maturity, about 0.5-1% of bone a year is lost in both sexes
- Women experience a phase of accelerated bone loss for 3-5 years after the menopause

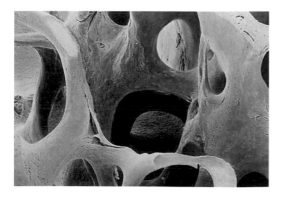
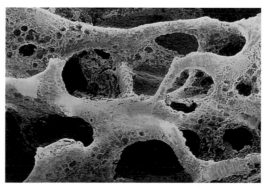

Comparison of structure of trabecular bone from healthy (left) and osteoporotic (right) subjects illustrating the architectural damage resulting from trabecular perforation

situations of increased bone turnover, for example, after the menopause, and the resulting loss of normal architecture leads to a disproportionate loss of strength for the amount of bone lost. Increased bone turnover is an independent predictor of fracture risk. This may reflect the increase in number of remodelling sites which can act as a stress riser and increase bone fragility.

Epidemiology

One in three women and one in twelve men are likely to sustain a fracture related to osteoporosis by the age of 90 years. The incidence of osteoporotic fractures is increasing more than expected from the ageing of the population. This may reflect changing patterns of exercise or diet in recent decades.

Classification of osteoporosis

Primary osteoporosis
Postmenopausal osteoporosis results from accelerated bone loss as a result of oestrogen deficiency. The increased rate of bone loss leads to predominant loss of trabecular bone and frequent trabecular perforation. This typically results in fractures of vertebral bodies and the distal forearm in the sixth and seventh decades of life.

Osteoporosis may also result from age-related reductions in bone that occur in both sexes because of remodelling imbalance. Less inequality between the rates of cortical and trabecular bone loss and the typical manifestation of fracture of the proximal femur is seen in elderly patients.

Secondary osteoporosis
Secondary osteoporosis accounts for up to 40% of cases of osteoporosis in women and 60% of cases in men.

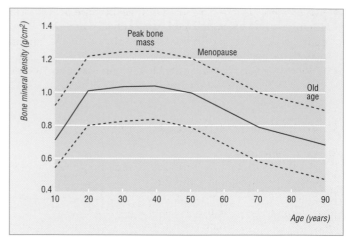

Association between age and bone mineral density of lumbar spine in women. Lines show mean (2 standard deviations)

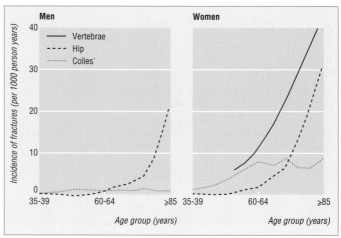

Incidence of osteoporotic fractures with age

Causes of secondary osteoporosis				
Endocrine	**Gastrointestinal**	**Rheumatological**	**Malignancy**	**Drugs**
• Thyrotoxicosis • Primary hyperparathyroidism • Cushing's syndrome • Hypogonadism	• Malabsorption syndrome, for example, Coeliac disease Partial gastrectomy • Liver disease, for example, Primary biliary cirrhosis	• Rheumatoid arthritis • Ankylosing spondylitis	• Multiple myeloma	• Corticosteroids • Heparin

Risk factors for osteoporotic fracture

Several risk factors for osteoporosis within populations are well established. These risk factors do not, however, have adequate sensitivity or specificity to identify people at risk, and measurement of bone mineral density is needed to quantify an individual's risk of fracture.

- *Hypogonadism*—Hypogonadism may be secondary to anorexia nervosa or excessive exercise, and it is an important cause of osteoporosis in men.
- *Smoking*—The effect of smoking may be mediated by smokers' tendency to have a lower body weight and female smokers' tendency to have an earlier menopause than non-smokers.
- *High alcohol consumption*—This may have a direct suppressive effect on bone formation, and it also may lead to hypogonadism.

Risk factors for osteoporosis
- Female sex
- Increasing age
- Early menopause (before age 45 years)
- Hypogonadism
- Smoking
- High alcohol intake
- Physical inactivity
- Low body mass index
- Heredity

Risk factors that act independently of bone mineral density
- Prevalent low trauma fracture, particularly vertebral fractures
- Family history, particularly of maternal hip fracture
- Current smoking habit
- Low body weight
- Increasing age

- *Low body mass index*—This increases risk because of diminished effects of mechanical stimuli and because conversion of androstenedione to oestrone occurs in adipose tissue in postmenopausal woman
- *Heredity*—Genetic factors probably account for up to 70% of the variability in peak bone mass.

Investigations for osteoporosis

Spinal radiographs
Up to half of vertebral fractures are asymptomatic and may be suspected from height loss and the development of kyphosis. They may also result from degenerative spinal disease, however, and radiographs of the thoracic and lumbar spine are important to differentiate fractures from degenerative changes. Osteopenia cannot be identified reliably from radiographic appearance, so bone densitometry is needed to quantify osteopenia, if suspected, and to monitor disease progression or response to treatment.

Bone densitometry
Bone density is usually measured by dual energy x ray absorptiometry—a technique that uses extremely low doses of ionising radiation to quantify bone mineral density accurately and precisely. Dual energy x ray absorptiometry of the spine and hip is the optimal clinical measurement for diagnosis. Measurement of bone density in peripheral skeletal sites with techniques such as quantitative ultrasound has useful predictive value for osteoporotic fractures, but appropriate intervention thresholds for these measurements remain uncertain, and they are probably not useful for monitoring responses to treatment.

Bone density is the major determinant of a person's risk of fracture. The predictive ability of bone density is comparable with that of blood pressure for determining the risk of cerebrovascular accident and of serum cholesterol for determining the risk of coronary thrombosis. The relative risk of fracture increases two- to threefold for each standard deviation decrease in bone density. Fracture risk is increased by the presence of independent risk factors.

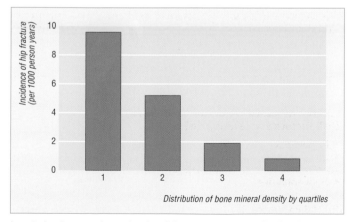

Association between bone density of the femoral neck and risk of hip fracture. The quarter of patients with lowest bone density had 8.5 times higher risk of fracture than the quarter with highest bone density

Indications for bone densitometry
Currently, no rationale exists for population screening of bone mineral density. Measurements should be targeted to individuals likely to be at increased risk of osteoporosis, in whom knowledge of bone mineral density will influence management. A number of categories may be defined in

---

Investigations

- Spinal radiographs
- Bone densitometry
- Screen for underlying causes
  Serum calcium, phosphate, alkaline phosphatase, parathyroid hormone, and creatinine
  24-hour urinary calcium and creatinine excretion
  Serum protein electrophoresis and urinary Bence Jones protein
  Thyroid stimulating hormone
  Full blood count and erythrocyte sedimentation rate
  Serum testosterone (in males)

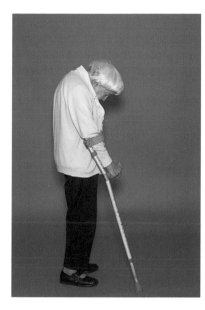

Height loss, kyphosis, and abdominal protrusion due to osteoporotic vertebral fractures in elderly woman

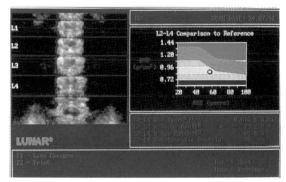

Bone density scan of the lumbar spine

Indications for bone densitometry

- Presence of strong risk factors

Oestrogen deficiency	Primary hyperparathyroidism
Premature menopause (age < 45 years)	Other disorders associated with osteoporosis
Prolonged secondary amenorrhoea (>1 year)	Anorexia nervosa
Primary hypogonadism	Malabsorption syndromes
Corticosteroid therapy	Post-transplantation
Maternal history of hip fracture	Chronic renal failure
Low body mass index (<19 kg/m²)	Hyperparathyroidism
	Prolonged immobilisation
	Cushing's syndrome

- Radiographic evidence of osteopenia and/or vertebral deformity
- Previous fragility fracture, particularly of hip spine or wrist
- Loss of height and thoracic kyphosis (after radiographic confirmation of vertebral deformities)

Prevention of osteoporosis

Optimising peak bone mass
- Exercise needs to be regular and weight bearing (such as walking or aerobics); excessive exercise may lead to bone loss
- Dietary calcium may be important, especially during growth
- Investigation and treatment of conditions predisposing to osteoporosis, for example, amenorrhoea
- Avoidance of smoking and excessive alcohol consumption

Reducing rate of bone loss
- Selective oestrogen receptor modulators
- Regular exercise
- Maintain calcium intake
- Avoidance of smoking and excessive alcohol consumption

whom bone mineral density measurement should be considered.

Individuals with a low trauma vertebral fracture or low bone mineral density for age should be investigated for underlying causes of osteoporosis. If access to bone densitometry is limited, it may be appropriate to treat individuals who have had previous low trauma fractures or who have other strong risk factors for fracture such as elderly people who need high dose corticosteroid therapy.

Prevention

Prevention should aim to increase peak bone mass and reduce the subsequent rate of bone loss.

Treatment

Treatment of established osteoporosis aims to alleviate the patient's symptoms and reduce the risk of further fractures. Currently available drugs act by reducing bone turnover to prevent further bone loss and are associated with a decrease in fracture risk of up to 50%.

Pain relief—Provided mainly by analgesics, but physical measures—such as hydrotherapy or transcutaneous nerve stimulators—may be useful adjuncts to treatment. The pain modulating effects of low dose antidepressants can be helpful, and many patients benefit from assessment at specialist pain clinics. The pain associated with fractures usually resolves within six months, but patients with vertebral fractures may need to be given long-term analgesia because of secondary degenerative disease. Techniques such as vertebroplasty currently are being evaluated for their potential to relieve the pain that occurs after vertebral fracture.

Drugs to reduce fracture risk—These act by inhibiting bone resorption and hence by reducing bone turnover. The reduction in fracture risk is related to the decreased rate of bone turnover and to small increases in bone mass that result from infilling of the remodelling space and increased secondary mineralisation. Drugs designed to increase bone mass by stimulating bone formation are in development. Recombinant parathyroid hormone injections, administered subcutaneously on a daily basis, have recently been licensed in the United Kingdom. Phase III studies with this treatment have shown decreases in vertebral fracture risk in the order of 70% over a year.

Treating underlying causes—Often leads to at least partial recovery of bone.

Preventing falls—Predisposing factors, such as postural hypotension or drowsiness due to drugs, should be eliminated where possible. Patients may benefit from physiotherapy to improve their balance and saving reflexes. Hip protectors, designed to absorb the impact of a fall onto the hip, have been shown to reduce the incidence of hip fracture among residents of nursing homes, although efficacy is limited by poor compliance. Patients should be provided with appropriate

Drugs to reduce fracture risk

Antiresorptive agents
- *Bisphosphonates*—Cyclical etidronate reduces bone loss from the spine and vertebral fracture risk in postmenopausal women with osteoporosis. Alendronate and risedronate both prevent bone loss from vertebral and non-vertebral sites and decrease the risk of spine and hip fractures. Poor absorption of these agents means they must be taken 30 minutes before breakfast (alendronate and risedronate) or on an empty stomach in the middle of a four-hour fast (cyclical etidronate). In an attempt to improve the convenience of the oral bisphosphonates, once weekly dosing is available for alendronate and is under development for risedronate. Phase III studies are looking at the use of potent bisphosphonates, which may be administered as an annual intravenous infusion
- The use of hormone replacement therapy is no longer thought to be appropriate in the management of osteoporosis unless it is needed to control climacteric symptoms, or in women under 50 who have undergone early menopause
- *Selective oestrogen receptor modulators*—These are synthetic agents that act as oestrogen agonists on bone and in relation to serum lipids, but without oestrogen-like stimulation of breast and endometrial tissues. Raloxifene reduces the risk of vertebral fracture but has not been shown to decrease the risk of non-vertebral fractures. Like hormone replacement therapy, raloxifene is associated with small increases in the number of thromboembolic events but conversely is associated with reduction in the number of new cases of breast cancer
- *Calcium (1000-1200 mg daily)*—This has a less marked effect on fracture reduction than the other antiresorptive agents but is usually well tolerated
- *Vitamin D (800 units daily) and calcium (1000-1200 mg daily)*—This has been shown to reduce hip fracture risk in the frail elderly and to cause a modest reduction in vertebral fracture risk in men and women over 65 years. It often is used as adjunctive therapy in combination with another antiresorptive agent
- *Calcium plus vitamin D*—A combination of calcium and vitamin D should be considered in all elderly patients who are housebound or in residential care
- *Calcitonin*—Calcitonin may be administered as subcutaneous injections or as a nasal preparation that is associated with fewer side effects. Calcitonin has been shown to reduce the risk of vertebral fracture. This agent has analgesic properties that may be useful in the acute management of vertebral fracture

Formation stimulating agents
- *Fluoride*—Dramatically increases bone mass, but evidence of fracture prevention is inconclusive and the therapeutic window is probably narrow. Consequently it is used rarely in the United Kingdom
- *Other agents*—Other agents, such as intermittent injections of recombinant parathyroid hormone have recently been licensed in the United Kingdom

walking aids, and an environmental assessment should be made of their accommodation to eliminate hazards such as loose rugs and cables. Visual assessment and treatment is also important. Assessment via specialised falls clinics may be appropriate.

Monitoring—The rationale for monitoring treatment response is that a proportion of patients fail to respond to treatment; in addition, compliance may improve when the patient sees the treatment working. The current standard measure used to monitor treatment response is dual energy x ray absorptiometry of the spine. Increasing evidence shows that biochemical markers of bone turnover may offer a more rapid assessment of treatment response—within 3-6 months. The decrease in bone turnover in response to antiresorptive agents may be a superior predictor of the decrease in fracture risk. These measurements are currently used only in some specialist centres, but assays for markers of bone resorption and formation are available on automated analysers. Further evaluation is needed to define the optimal protocol for measuring markers before they can be used routinely.

Education

An important part of the management of osteoporosis is education and support of the patient, their carers, and their family. Groups such as the National Osteoporosis Society have a vital role in this area.

National Osteoporosis Society (NOS)
Camerton
Bath BA2 OPJ
Tel: 01761 471771 (for general enquiries)
0845 4500230 (for medical enquiries)

Further reading

- Barlow D, ed. *Osteoporosis. Clinical guidelines for prevention and treatment.* London: Royal College of Physicians, 1999
- Royal College of Physicians. *Glucocorticoid-induced osteoporosis. Guidelines for prevention and treatment.* London: Royal College of Physicians, 2002
- National Osteoporosis Foundation. Osteoporosis: review of the evidence for prevention, diagnosis and treatment and cost-effectiveness analysis. *Osteoporosis Int* 1998;8:1-88S

11 Rheumatoid arthritis: clinical features and diagnosis

Mohammed Akil, Kiran Veerapen

Rheumatoid arthritis is the most common inflammatory arthritis and is an important cause of disability, morbidity, and mortality. Disease modifying therapy has a positive impact on disease progression, but complete remission is rare.

Rheumatoid arthritis causes early joint damage and functional limitation, both of which progress slowly with time. Ten years from onset, work-related disability is present in about half of the patients. Estimates of reduction in life expectancy range from three to ten years. In subsets of patients with poor prognostic markers, mortality rates are comparable to stage IV Hodgkin's disease or triple vessel coronary artery disease. Cardiovascular disease, complications of rheumatoid arthritis, and gastropathy induced by non-steroidal anti-inflammatory drugs are important causes of the excess mortality. Patients with rheumatoid arthritis may be offered life insurance on the basis of loaded premiums.

Some studies suggest that rheumatoid arthritis is declining in frequency and severity. The expression of rheumatoid arthritis is largely homogenous, and the pattern of joint involvement is modified by environmental and possibly genetic factors. Rheumatoid arthritis associated extra-articular disease has been consistently less common in Asians and Africans than in Caucasians.

Rheumatoid arthritis occurs worldwide with variable incidence and severity

Effect of rheumatoid arthritis on the hand—early changes

Effect of rheumatoid arthritis on the hand—early changes

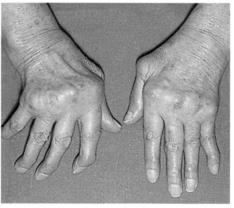

Effect of rheumatoid arthritis on the hand—later deformity

Cause

The cause of rheumatoid arthritis remains unclear, but evidence shows a genetic predisposition to the disease. The genetic contribution in rheumatoid arthritis is around 15-20%. It does not affect the clinical expression of rheumatoid arthritis. The risk of rheumatoid arthritis in first degree relatives is almost double that among the general population.

The presence of major histocompatibility complex class II allele human leucocyte antigen-DR4 is more common among patients with rheumatoid arthritis who are white, and other ethnic groups have different associations. This apparently confusing finding can be explained by the presence of a shared epitope in the third hypervariable region of the human leucocyte antigen-DRB 1 chain.

The concept that rheumatoid arthritis is triggered by an infection in a genetically susceptible individual remains popular, but no specific infection has been unequivocally implicated.

Onset and evolution

Rheumatoid arthritis is a rare disease in men under the age of 30 years. The incidence rises to peak at 60-70 years. In women, the prevalence of disease increases from the mid 20s to a fairly constant level at 45-75 years and a broad peak at 65-75 years.

Rheumatoid arthritis often begins in the post-partum period but links with physical trauma or psychological stress are difficult to establish. The typical onset is insidious and polyarticular, with symmetrical involvement of the metacarpophalangeal, proximal interphalangeal, wrist, and metatarsophalangeal joints. More acute onset with large joint involvement is more common in elderly patients. Less common patterns of onset are a persistent monoarthritis or oligoarthritis. The distribution may sometimes be asymmetrical. Occasionally a polymyalgia-like presentation is seen. Up to half of patients with palindromic rheumatism later develop typical rheumatoid arthritis, which is often accompanied by conversion to seropositivity for rheumatoid factor. The disease is usually polyphasic and progressive, but it may be monophasic or episodic in nature.

The pathological spectrum of rheumatoid arthritis spans across early disease, when joints exhibit active synovitis without structural damage, to late disease, when the joints may be mechanically damaged, malaligned, and unstable, without persistent active synovitis. Inflammation of other extra-articular synovial structures, such as tendon sheaths and their consequent attenuation, shortening, displacement, rupture, or nodularity, add to disability and are responsible for some of the characteristic rheumatoid deformities—ulnar deviation of the fingers, z deformity of the thumb, and swan neck and boutonnière deformities. The most serious long-term disability is associated with damage to the large weight-bearing joints.

Involvement at specific sites

The disease may start in a few joints, but often most joints become involved with time.

Cervical spine—The cervical spine's discovertebral joints are often affected and symptomatic (25-33%). This may lead to atlantoaxial subluxation or less often subluxation at lower levels, with subsequent compression of the spinal cord. The most common symptom of subluxation is pain that radiates up into the occiput. Anterior subluxation is best detected in a lateral x ray examination of the cervical spine during flexion. Instability at C1-C2 can be gauged by measuring the change in distance between the posterior rim of the arch of atlas and anterior margin of dens between the lateral extension and flexion views. Many patients have a stable deformity without neurological deficit.

Thoracic and lumbar apophyseal joints—These are lined by synovium but are rarely involved in the rheumatoid process.

Axial joints—The temporomandibular, cricoarytenoid, sternoclavicular, and interossicle joints may be affected.

Shoulder—Intermittent shoulder pain may precede onset of rheumatoid arthritis. In advanced disease, glenohumeral destruction with upward subluxation of the humerus is seen.

Unusual patterns of onset of rheumatoid arthritis

- Palindromic
- Monoarthritic
- Symmetrical
- Polymyalgic
- Oligoarthritic

Site involvement of rheumatoid arthritis

- Cervical spine
- Thoracic and lumbar apophyseal joints
- Axial joints
- Shoulder
- Elbow
- Wrist
- Hand
- Hip
- Knee
- Hind foot
- Fore foot

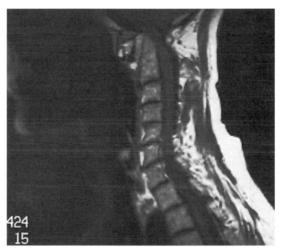

Magnetic resonance image of cervical spine showing spinal cord compression at C1 and C2

Symptoms of subluxation

- Pain that radiates into occiput
- Paraesthesiae
- Sudden deterioration in hand function
- Sensory loss
- Abnormal gait
- Urinary retention or incontinence

Causes of impaired hand function in rheumatoid arthritis

- Active synovitis
- Joint deformity
- Rupture of tendon, tenosynovitis, trigger finger
- Carpal tunnel syndrome
- Mononeuritis
- Compression of nerve root at T1
- Compression of spinal cord

Elbow—Clinical damage with some loss of pronation, supination, or extension is present in up to half the patients with longstanding disease.

Wrist—Up to two thirds of patients with longstanding disease have involvement of the wrist, which contributes to poor hand function and grip strength. Tenosynovitis of anterior tendons may lead to carpal tunnel entrapment.

Hand—The metacarpophalangeal, proximal interphalangeal, and thumb interphalangeal joints often are all involved. Distal interphalangeal joints are not involved in isolation. Flexor tenosynovitis with thickening, nodularity, and triggering contributes to functional impairment.

Hip—Hip pain is uncommon in early disease, but this underestimates the level of hip involvement, which may be present in one third of patients with early disease.

Knee—Overall, 50% of patients develop damage in the knees with longstanding disease. Weakness of the quadriceps muscle develops early and contributes to knee instability. Effusion of the knee may produce a popliteal (Baker's) cyst. This may rupture to cause pain and swelling in the calf that mimics deep vein thrombosis.

Hind foot—Inflammation of the ankle, subtalar, and midtarsal joints, along with the Achilles tendon, surrounding bursae, and the medial and lateral ankle tendons, are responsible for pain and deformity in this region. The classical flat everted foot of rheumatoid arthritis is a result of subtalar joint arthritis.

Fore foot—In Caucasian patients, pain and tenderness in the fore foot is very common. Weight bearing on the tender metatarsophalangeal heads causes a sensation of "walking on pebbles." Hallux valgus is common and probably a result of tight, squeezing footwear. Hallux varus and toe splaying are also found in populations where open footwear is worn routinely.

Extra-articular manifestations

Some extra-articular features are a result of vasculitis, granuloma, or nodule formation and are related to high levels of rheumatoid factor. Others are a consequence of mechanical effects of joint disease.

Fatigue and malaise are common features of active rheumatoid arthritis, but fever is uncommon.

Rheumatoid nodules—These affect about one fifth of Caucasian patients and less than 10% of Asian patients. They may occur anywhere but are most common at sites of pressure, notably the extensor surfaces of the forearms.

Vascular lesions—Disease of small blood vessels may be caused by deposition of immune complex in the vascular walls. This can lead to digital infarction, large skin ulcers, and mononeuritis multiplex.

Renal disease—This is rare but may occur as a result of amyloidosis, which presents as proteinuria. More often, renal abnormalities are a result of the use of non-steroidal anti-inflammatory drugs or disease modifying antirheumatic drugs.

Eye complications

Sjögren's syndrome—Sicca complex results in dry gritty eyes with slight redness but normal vision. Schirmer test, which measures wetting of a strip of sterilised filter paper, confirms diagnosis.

Episcleritis—This results in ocular irritation with nodules. Vision is normal.

Scleritis—This causes severe pain and occasionally reduces vision. Diffuse or nodular redness is seen; the end stage of the condition is healing, when atrophy forms a bluish-grey sclera.

Extra-articular complications

- Fatigue
- Malaise
- Rheumatoid nodules
- Vascular lesions
- Renal disease
- Osteoporosis
- Ocular
  Sjögren's syndrome
  Episcleritis
  Scleritis
- Haematological
  Anaemia
  Neutrophilia
  Thrombocytosis
  Felty's syndrome
- Neurological
  Entrapment of peripheral nerves
  Mononeuritis multiplex
  Peripheral neuropathy
- Pulmonary
  Asymptomatic bilateral pleural effusions
  Rheumatoid nodules
  Interstitial disease
  Bronchiolitis obliterans organising pneumonia
- Cardiac
  Pericarditis
  Myocardial granuloma or nodules
  Myocardial infarction

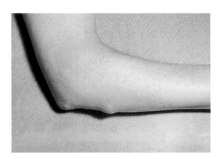
Rheumatoid nodule

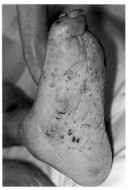
Rheumatoid vasculitis

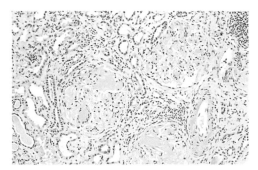
Renal amyloid (Congo red stain)

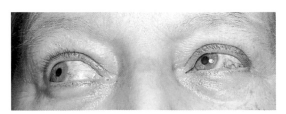
Scleritis associated with rheumatoid arthritis

Haematological complications

Anaemia is present in more than half of patients with rheumatoid arthritis, particularly those with active disease. Neutrophilia may be seen with active disease, intercurrent infection, and corticosteroid use. Thrombocytosis occurs with active disease or after a bleed. Felty's syndrome—a combination of seropositive rheumatoid arthritis (often with relatively inactive synovitis), splenomegaly, and neutropenia—is associated with serious infections, vasculitis (leg ulcers, mononeuritis), anaemia, thrombocytopenia, and lymphadenopathy.

Neurological complications

These include entrapment of peripheral nerves (carpal tunnel, ulnar, lateral popliteal, tarsal, etc), mononeuritis multiplex, peripheral neuropathy (either associated with the disease or caused by drugs), and compression of nerve roots and the spinal cord, which occur with mechanical complications of the disease in the cervical region.

Pulmonary

Asymptomatic bilateral pleural effusions are not uncommon in men with seropositive disease. Rheumatoid nodules are found in less than 1% of patients and may cavitate. They need to be differentiated from primary and metastatic malignancy. Interstitial disease occurs in 1-5% of cases and generally progresses slowly, but it may remain stable or even improve over the years. Bronchiolitis obliterans organising pneumonia presents as a subacute interstitial pneumonia and responds to treatment with steroids.

Bone and osteoporosis

Osteoporosis both in the axial and appendicular sites is common. It is a result of the inflammatory process, immobility and use of corticosteroids. Fracture risk in patients with rheumatoid arthritis is twice that in the general population.

Assessment

History

Assessment of a patient with rheumatoid arthritis involves taking a careful history of pain, stiffness after inactivity, joint swelling, and fatigue. Knowledge of the patient's socioeconomic circumstances and presence of anxiety or depression are useful.

Prognostic factors

Prediction of the outcome of rheumatoid arthritis in an individual patient at disease outset is difficult. The presence of indicators of poor outcome help identify patients who need aggressive therapy.

Clinical evaluation

Signs common to many joints are warmth and tenderness on palpation. Muscle wasting around the joints is frequently evident. Swelling may be boggy when a result of synovitis, fluctuant as a result of an effusion, or bony as a result of malalignment. Instability, which often precedes malalignment (subluxation or dislocation), may be detected in the peripheral joints. Loss of range of movement may be reversible when it is a result of synovial swelling or effusion, or permanent when it is due to malalignment and capsular contracture. Swelling, tenderness, or nodularity of the periarticular structures contribute to pain.

Causes of anaemia in rheumatoid arthritis

- Anaemia of chronic disease
- Iron deficiency—blood loss caused by non-steroidal anti-inflammatory drugs
- Suppression of bone marrow function—caused by sulfasalazine, penicillamine, gold, and cytotoxic drugs
- Folate deficiency—caused by sulfasalazine, methotrexate
- Vitamin B-12 deficiency—caused by associated pernicious anaemia
- Haemolysis—caused by sulfasalazine and dapsone
- Felty's syndrome

Cardiac manifestations—Pericarditis is the most common cardiac manifestation and may be recurrent or constrictive in some patients. Myocardial granuloma or nodules may be responsible for conduction defects and occasionally are found on myocardial valves and at the root of the aorta. Myocardial infarction may be a result of coronary vasculitis

Cardiovascular morbidity and mortality are increased in rheumatoid arthritis

---

Factors associated with poor prognosis in patients with rheumatoid arthritis

- Many active joints at onset
- Extra-articular manifestations
- Poor scores on functional assessment
- High levels of rheumatoid factor
- Presence of human leucocyte antigen-DR4
- Early evidence of radiological erosions
- Low socioeconomic status
- Early and late age at onset

Serial records of pain, stiffness, swollen joint, and functional impairment are useful to gauge the disease's activity or impact

Investigations

No single test can diagnose rheumatoid arthritis. Investigations are used largely to support the clinical diagnosis, and negative results do not exclude a diagnosis of rheumatoid arthritis. Investigations in early disease aim to show raised inflammatory markers and exclude other differential diagnoses. Immune abnormalities, including the presence of rheumatoid factor, should be sought. The American College of Rheumatology criteria for classification of rheumatoid arthritis are used in diagnosis predominantly for research purposes.

Differential diagnosis of rheumatoid arthritis

- Psoriatic arthritis or other seronegative spondylarthropathy
- Primary nodal osteoarthritis
- Polyarticular gout
- Other connective tissue diseases
- Calcium pyrophosphate deposition disease

American Rheumatism Association 1987 revised criteria for the classification of rheumatoid arthritis

Diagnosis of rheumatoid arthritis needs four of seven of the following criteria. In criteria 1-4, the joint signs or symptoms must be continuous for at least six weeks.
1 Morning stiffness of duration longer than one hour for longer than six weeks
2 Arthritis of three or more joint areas* Soft tissue swelling or effusion lasting longer than six weeks
3 Arthritis of hand joints (wrist, metacarpophalangeal joints, or proximal interphalangeal joints) lasting longer than six weeks
4 Symmetric arthritis* in at least one area lasting longer than six weeks
5 Rheumatoid nodules, as observed by a doctor
6 Serum rheumatoid factor, as assessed by a method positive in less than 5% of control subjects
7 Radiographic changes, as seen on anteroposterior radiograph of wrists and hands

*Possible areas: proximal interphalangeal joints, metacarpophalangeal joints, wrist, elbow, knee, ankle, and metatarsophalangeal joints
(Observed by a physician)

Other causes of positive test for rheumatoid factor

- Other connective tissue diseases
- Viral infections
- Leprosy
- Leishmaniasis
- Subacute bacterial endocarditis
- Tuberculosis
- Liver diseases
- Sarcoidosis
- Mixed essential cryoglobulinemia

Laboratory findings in rheumatoid arthritis

- Anaemia—normochromic or hypochromic, normocytic (if microcytic consider iron deficiency)
- Thrombocytosis
- Raised erythrocyte sedimentation rate
- Raised Creactive protein concentration
- Raised ferritin concentration as acute phase protein
- Low serum iron concentration
- Low total iron binding capacity
- Raised serum globulin concentrations
- Raised serum alkaline phosphatase activity
- Presence of rheumatoid factor

Immune abnormalities

Rheumatoid factors are anti-immunoglobulins.

Immunoglobulin M (rheumatoid factor) is detected with the Rose-Waaler assay, but it is neither universally present in rheumatoid arthritis nor specific for it—it is found in the sera of 70-80% of patients with rheumatoid arthritis. Such patients may carry rheumatoid factors of other isotypes. Extra-articular features are more common in patients with high concentrations of rheumatoid factor, but it is a poor guide to the severity of joint disease. Antinuclear antibodies are found in some patients.

Indicators of acute phase response

Raised erythrocyte sedimentation rate (or plasma viscosity) and the presence of acute phase proteins such as C reactive protein reflect the severity of acute inflammation. A reduction in levels of serum albumin and haemoglobin may also confirm the presence of active inflammation.

Liver function

Serum concentrations of transaminases and alkaline phosphatase may be raised moderately in patients with active disease. This may confound changes related to disease modifying antirheumatic drugs.

Radiography

X ray examinations—The standard means for assessing erosive damage. Erosions typical of rheumatoid arthritis develop within three years of the start of disease in > 90% of patients who ultimately develop them. Early erosions may be seen in the metacarpophalangeal and metatarsophalangeal joints and in the wrists. Erosions are marginal and accompanied by periarticular osteoporosis. Later, joint space narrowing, subluxation, and secondary osteoarthritic changes are evident.

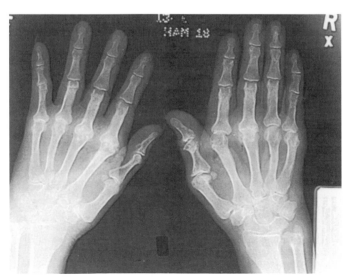

Radiograph of hands showing rheumatoid erosions

Computed tomography—Used to image bony lesions in the axial skeleton—the temporomandibular and sternoclavicular joints.

Magnetic resonance imaging—Allows good visualisation of the soft tissues and bony structures and is very useful in imaging of the spine.

Ultrasonography—A cheap technique that defines superficial soft tissue lesions—for example, Baker's cysts, tenosynovitis, and bursitis.

Joint scintigraphy—Areas with increased pick up of radionuclide show hyperaemia and synovial inflammation—useful for detecting stress fractures.

Further reading

- Lindqvist E, Eberhardt K. Mortality in rheumatoid arthritis patients with disease onset in the 1980s. *Ann Rheum Dis* 1999;58:11-14
- Cooper NJ. Economic burden of rheumatoid arthritis: a systematic review. *Rheumatology* 2000;39:28-33
- Lee DM, Weinblatt ME. Rheumatoid arthritis (review). *Lancet* 2001;358:903-11

With Acknowledgments to Dr Edward Roddy, Specialist Registrar in Rheumatology, Mid-Trent, for additional suggestions for further reading.

12 Rheumatoid arthritis: treatment

Mohammed Akil, Kiran Veerapen

Except for the mildest cases, rheumatoid arthritis can only be managed adequately by a multidisciplinary team approach. Most people with rheumatoid arthritis cope better if they understand their condition and have realistic expectations of the benefits and disadvantages of treatment. Rheumatology clinical nurse specialists play a vital role by educating patients about their disease and drug therapy, monitoring drugs used in rheumatoid arthritis, and differentiating minor or unrelated symptoms from those that need action.

Physical therapy

Local measures such as heat, cold, and ultrasound may be used to reduce pain. They are used generally as part of a rehabilitation programme of exercises designed to improve muscle strength and encourage mobility in affected joints.

Few of the individual techniques used in physiotherapy and occupational therapy have been subject to controlled trials, but three is no doubt that experienced therapists who are skilled in handling atrophied, inflamed, and stiff tissues and are familiar with the problems faced by patients with arthritis are of irreplaceable value in treatment and rehabilitation.

Surgery for rheumatoid arthritis

Although synovectomy may slow progression of damage for a relatively short period, it does not alter the outcome. These procedures are becoming relatively uncommon among "arthritis surgeons," who have taken on the role of reconstruction.

The patient must be part of the decision making process, which also should include the rheumatologist and surgeon. The patient thus should have a realistic understanding of the procedure. The timing of surgery is crucial. For example, fore foot arthroplasty should usually precede knee or hip arthroplasty, as the risk of infection is minimised.

Medication

Non-steroidal anti-inflammatory drugs

These drugs provide symptomatic relief but do not modify the course of the disease. In the mildest cases they may be used alone, but more often they are used in combination with disease modifying drugs. The individual response to the different non-steroidal anti-inflammatory drugs varies somewhat and several drugs may be tried before a suitable one is identified.

By inhibiting the synthesis of cyclooxygenase enzymes, non-steroidal anti-inflammatory drugs reduce production of inflammatory prostaglandin. Two main isoforms of cyclooxygenase exist: cyclooxygenase I and cyclooxygenase II. The anti-inflammatory effects of non-steroidal anti-inflammatory drugs are achieved through inhibition of cyclooxygenase II. Inhibition of cyclooxygenase I is responsible for the toxicity of these drugs, especially their gastric side effects. Newer

---

Therapeutic goals in rheumatoid arthritis

1 Symptomatic relief
2 Preservation of function
3 Prevention of structural damage and deformity
4 Maintenance of the patient's normal lifestyle
5 Increase function

Aims of physical therapy for rheumatoid arthritis

Physiotherapy
- Patient education
- Pain reduction
- Joint mobilisation to minimise deformity
- Muscle strengthening and prevention of disuse atrophy

Occupational therapy
- Patient education
- Joint protection
- Analysis and improvement of function with:
    Exercise
    Use of aids and appliances
- Provision of splints

Podiatry
- Local re-distribution to avoid callus
- Provision of customised orthoses and insoles to improve toe and foot posture and function
- Provision of foot care to prevent local infection

Orthotics
- Provision of specialised footwear
- Provision of orthoses

Surgery for rheumatoid arthritis

Aims of surgery
- Pain relief
- Restoration of function

Indications for urgent surgery
- Septic arthritis
- Tendon rupture
- Spinal cord and nerve decompression

Corrective surgical procedures
- Cervical fusion for subluxation
- Arthrodesis
- Replacement arthroplasty
- Excision arthroplasty

Two main isoforms of cyclooxygenase

Cyclooxygenase I
- Constitutively expressed in most tissues
- Responsible for production of prostaglandins important for homoeostatic functions, such as maintaining integrity of gastric mucosa

Cyclooxygenase II
- Expressed during inflammation
- Responsible for production of inflammatory prostaglandins

non-steroidal anti-inflammatory drugs selectively inhibit cyclooxygenase II and have been shown in clinical trials to be as effective as standard non-steroidal anti-inflammatory drugs.

All non-steroidal anti-inflammatory drugs are associated with adverse events. Some are relatively specific to a drug, such as headaches with indomethacin, but others are generic to the group, especially gastrointestinal and renal side effects. Of particular concern is the propensity of non-steroidal anti-inflammatory drugs, including the cyclooxygenase II selective agents, to cause gastrointestinal toxicity.

Gastrointestinal side effects

Toxicity includes life-threatening perforations, ulcers, and bleeds. The incidence seems to be much less, however, with cyclooxygenase II selective agents such as celecoxib, rofecoxib, etoricoxib, valdecoxib, and meloxicam. They should be preferred to standard non-steroidal anti-inflammatory drugs in patients at high risk of developing serious gastrointestinal toxicity.

When used with standard non-steroidal anti-inflammatory drugs, histamine-2 blockers reduce the risk of duodenal ulceration but have little protective effects against gastric ulcers. The prostaglandin E1 analogue misoprostol offers protection against gastric and duodenal ulcers but its use is limited by the high incidence of diarrhoea and abdominal pain. Proton pump inhibitors reduce the risk of gastric and duodenal toxicity. No evidence justifies their use with cyclooxygenase II selective inhibitors to further reduce potential gastrointestinal toxicity.

Renal side effects

Non-steroidal anti-inflammatory drugs should be used with caution in patients with renal failure, cardiac failure, or uncontrolled hypertension so as to avoid decompensation due to renal prostanoid blockade. Interstitial nephritis may present idiosyncratically rather than being linked to cyclooxygenase inhibition. Cyclooxygenase II selective inhibitors offer no advantage over standard non-steroidal anti-inflammatory drugs with respect to renal toxicity. Concomitant administration of non-steroidal anti-inflammatory drugs with anticoagulants is best avoided where possible.

Pregnancy

Administration of non-steroidal anti-inflammatory drugs in the later stages of pregnancy delays the onset and increases the duration of labour. It may lead to premature closure of ductus arteriosus in utero and possibly to persistent pulmonary hypertension of the newborn. Non-steroidal anti-inflammatory drugs in usual therapeutic doses are probably safe to use in lactating mothers with the exception of aspirin, which may increase the risk of Reye's syndrome in children.

Simple analgesia

Paracetamol, dextropropoxyphene, and codeine are used for simple pain relief. The choice is not critical but depends on patient preference. The use of stronger narcotic analgesics should be avoided.

Corticosteroids

Corticosteroids can be used in three main ways:

1 To settle a flare up
2 As an adjunct to slower acting second-line drugs
3 As regular treatment.

The use of higher doses (>7.5 mg daily) should be avoided in the absence of systemic complications. Continual corticosteroid therapy exacerbates the local and systemic

---

Examples of cyclooxygenase II selective agents

- Celecoxib
- Rofecoxib
- Etoricoxib
- Valdecoxib
- Meloxicam

Side effects of non-steroidal anti-inflammatory drugs

Gastrointestinal
- Dyspepsia, gastritis
- Gastric or duodenal ulceration
- Diarrhoea
- Hepatitis

Neurological
- Headache, dizziness
- Tinnitus
- Confusion
- Aseptic meningitis

Renal
- Precipitation of acute renal failure
- Haematuria
- Nephrotic syndrome
- Papillary necrosis
- Interstitial nephritis

Haematological
- Neutropenia
- Thrombocytopenia
- Aplastic anaemia
- Haemolytic anaemia

Respiratory
- Asthma
- Pneumonitis

Cardiovascular
- Oedema
- Hypertension
- Heart failure

Ovarian
- Delayed hypersensitivity reactions

Factors associated with high risk of gastrointestinal toxicity

- Age ≥ 65 years
- Previous history of peptic ulcer (or complication)
- Concomitant use of steroids and anticoagulants
- Presence of co-morbidity (cardiovascular disease, renal and hepatic impairment, diabetes and hypertension)
- Requirement for the prolonged use of maximum recommended doses of standard non-steroidal anti-inflammatory drugs

---

Uses of corticosteroids in rheumatoid arthritis

1 Intra-articular steroids can be helpful in settling a flare up
   - Long-acting (depot) steroids triamcinolone or methylprednisolone usually used for injection of large joints
   - Hydrocortisone or prednisolone advisable for superficial joints or flexor tendon sheaths, because of a lower incidence of subcutaneous and skin atrophy
2 Bolus intravenous or intramuscular corticosteroids as adjunct to the slower acting second-line drugs
   - May be used during flare up, although more often used in management of some of the systemic complications of rheumatoid arthritis
   - Potential hazards include avascular bone necrosis, spread of systemic sepsis, and cardiac arrhythmias
3 Regular daily oral corticosteroids often used to treat rheumatoid arthritis
   - Although controversy persists, low doses of corticosteroids, in combination with disease modifying drugs, have been shown to reduce rate of progression of joint damage

osteopenia that accompanies active and chronic rheumatoid arthritis. No dose avoids risk. Assessment of other risk factors and bone mineral density and, if necessary, the use of prophylactic therapy is important when systemic steroids are used on a long-term basis.

Disease modifying antirheumatic drugs

These drugs play a key role in the treatment of rheumatoid arthritis. They should be used early (as soon as the diagnosis is made) and continuously. The logic has rested largely on recognition of the serious long-term outcome of rheumatoid arthritis and thus the need to intervene early with most effective drugs and not wait for the development of joint damage.

All disease modifying antirheumatic drugs are potentially toxic and regular monitoring for toxicity is necessary. There is considerable variation among rheumatologists in monitoring schedules, and those given below reflect the experience and practice of the authors.

Individual patients differ in the aggressiveness of their disease and its concomitant structural damage, and the effect of their disease on their quality of life. These factors should be examined when considering disease modifying antirheumatic drugs in addition to the toxicity of the drugs.

Combination therapy

Combinations of disease modifying antirheumatic drugs in combination can improve disease control without increasing the risk of toxicity. The commonest combination is sulfasalazine, methotrexate, and hydroxychloroquine. Other combinations have been used. It is a common practice to combine disease modifying antirheumatic drugs with a small dose of oral steroid.

Examples of disease modifying antirheumatic drugs

- Methotrexate
- Leflunomide
- Sulfasalazine
- Hydroxychloroquine
- D-Penicillamine
- Gold therapy
- Azathioprine
- Cyclosporin
- Cyclophosphamide
- Combination therapy

Leflunomide

- Leflunomide is used increasingly as a second choice disease modifying antirheumatic drug. It is given as an oral dose of 20 mg daily (occasionally 10 mg). A loading dose of 100 mg daily for three days can hasten the onset of action. Leflunomide has similar efficacy to methotrexate. Adverse effects include diarrhoea, hypertension, abnormal liver function, leucopenia, rash, and hair loss.
- Like methotrexate, leflunomide is teratogenic in animals and should not be used by women or men wishing to have a family. The washout period is two years. This can be shortened to a few weeks by administration of cholestyramine or activated charcoal.
- The manufacturers suggest fortnightly blood counts and liver function test at six months then two months.

Hydroxychloroquine

- Antimalarials used in the management of rheumatoid arthritis are less effective but safer than some disease modifying antirheumatic drugs. Retinopathy is the major serious side effect and this is more common with chloroquine than hydroxychloroquine. Ophthalmic review is preferable.

Gold therapy

- Injectable gold (myocrisin) has symptomatic benefits for some patients with rheumatoid arthritis but the likelihood of them remaining on it in the long term is modest.
- The most common reactions are skin rashes. Not all rashes caused by gold therapy need permanent cessation of therapy.
- Proteinuria can be the precursor to serious renal problems and when persistent it should be investigated and gold withheld.
- Blood dyscrasia is a potentially lethal problem. The data sheet recommends that a blood count should be obtained before each injection. This is not always practical, and a large number of rheumatologists differ from this view, although they do agree that regular blood monitoring is important.
- Auranofin is an oral preparation of gold. Diarrhoea is more common, but it is not a major problem although it often leads to discontinuation of the drug. It is less effective than injectable gold and the two agents should not be regarded as interchangeable drugs. Regular blood and urine monitoring are needed.
- Long-term use of gold causes a greyish blue discolouration of the skin (cysiasis) that can be confused with cyanosis.

Methotrexate

- Methotrexate is given in small once weekly oral or injectable doses. It has become the disease modifying antirheumatic drugs of choice in most centres. It is relatively cheap and very well tolerated. The usual weekly dose is 10-20 mg (30 mg if tolerated).
- The most common side effect is nausea, which usually is not severe and may settle. More serious side effects include bone marrow suppression and alveolitis. A rise in serum transaminases is occasionally seen, but the risk of hepatic fibrosis and cirrhosis seems to be very rare. This drug should be avoided in patients with existing liver diseases or those who have a more than modest alcohol intake.
- It is important to avoid the use of cotrimoxazole and trimethoprim, as they can precipitate blood dyscrasia—probably because of folic acid deficiency in patients who take methotrexate.
- It is advisable to use regular folic acid supplements in all patients on methotrexate.
- As with other immunosuppressants, including steroids, the risk of herpes zoster and chickenpox is increased, and exposure to infected patients should be avoided.
- Women should not get pregnant and men should not father children while taking methotrexate and for 3-6 months after stopping the drug. Adequate contraception should be used.
- A chest x ray should be obtained before treatment is started with methotrexate. Blood count and liver function should be checked at baseline and then every two weeks for two months, monthly for six months, and then every two months.

Sulfasalazine

- About 60% of patients continue taking sulfasalazine after three years, with 15% withdrawals because of toxicity.
- The usual approach is to give 0.5 or 1.0 g/day increasing over
- 3-4 weeks to the maintenance dose of 2.0 g/day. This may be further increased to 2.5-3.0 g if required (and tolerated) after three months on 2 g/day.
- Adverse effects include nausea, headache, and abdominal discomfort and the incidence of such side effects is probably reduced by the use of enteric-coated tablets. Skin rash is an occasional problem, and the drug should not be used in patients who are allergic to sulphonamides. Desensitisation is possible through the use of very small but increasing doses that come in a special pack.
- Bone marrow suppression and hepatitis are among the more serious side effects and are more common in the first six months. It is advised to check the blood count and liver function before starting, at monthly intervals for three months, and then once every 3-6 months.
- Other side effects include reversible oligospermia and, as sulfasalazine is excreted in most body fluids, yellow discolouration of urine and soft contact lenses.

D-Penicillamine

- D-Penicillamine has a wide variety of potential side effects. A metallic taste in the mouth with nausea is a frequent early problem, but it resolves with continued use. Skin rashes, bone marrow suppression, and proteinuria are much more serious.
- Regular monitoring of blood and urine should be at monthly intervals initially and is often reduced thereafter; however, toxicity may intervene at any stage.

Cyclosporin

- Cyclosporin is expensive and potentially toxic with a 40% risk of renal impairment and hypertension. It is best reserved for resistant patients. Other adverse effects include gingival hyperplasia, tremor, and hirsutism.
- The usual dose is 2-3 mg/kg/day. It does not cause bone marrow suppression. Regular monitoring of blood pressure and serum creatinine is important.

Biological drugs

These drugs target a specific proinflammatory molecule. The first to be introduced have been those that inhibit the actions of tumour necrosis factor alpha or interleukin 1.

These drugs are recommended for patients who have continuing disease activity that has not responded adequately to at least two disease modifying antirheumatic drugs. A central "biological registry" has been set up in the United Kingdom and other European countries. Information on dosage, outcome, and toxicity are regularly circulated to participating clinicians, as long-term toxicity is not yet established.

About two thirds of patients respond to these therapies. Treatment should be withdrawn after three months if patients fail to respond.

These drugs are administered by intravenous or subcutaneous routes, and they have a rapid onset of action. They reduce inflammation, improve function, and prevent structural damage.

The main adverse effect is an increase in the rate of infection. Upper respiratory infections are the most common. Serious infections are rare and these drugs should not be given to patients who have active infection or are at high risk of infection (chronic leg ulcers, previous history of tuberculosis, recurrent chest infection, septic arthritis within the last 12 months, or indwelling urinary catheter).

Demyelination has been reported in some patients with multiple sclerosis who received anti-tumour necrosis factor therapy. A theoretical increased risk of malignancy exists, but this has not been shown to be the case so far. They should not be used in patients with a history of malignancy of less than 10 years, with the exception of basal cell carcinoma.

Women who are pregnant or breastfeeding should not receive biological drugs. Effective contraception must be practised.

Complementary medicine and rheumatoid arthritis

Since there is no cure for rheumatoid arthritis to be offered by the conventional aspects of management mentioned above, many patients turn to complementary medicine. Some of these approaches to management are getting closer to the practice of orthodox medicine. Patients may respond to advertisements in the lay press for supplements to their diet and yet others turn to homeopathy and more recently to reflexology or iridology.

Cyclophosphamide

- Cyclophosphamide is used mainly to treat systemic vasculitis associated with rheumatoid arthritis. It rarely is used to treat resistant synovitis. In addition to the risks encountered with other immunosuppressants, long-term use of cyclophosphamide is associated with gonadal failure, haemorrhagic cystitis, and haematological malignancies.

Azathioprine

- Azathioprine is used for synovitis and systemic complications of rheumatoid arthritis. The main initial limiting factor is nausea. Regular blood monitoring is necessary for early detection of bone marrow suppression or derangement of liver function. The usual dose is 2.5 mg/kg/day.

Etanercept

- Etanercept is a recombinant human tumour necrosis factor receptor fusion protein that acts competitively to inhibit binding of tumour necrosis factor to its cell surface receptor.
- It is administered by subcutaneous injection at a dose of 25 mg twice a week.
- Injection site reaction is the most common adverse effect.

Infliximab

- Infliximab is a chimeric (partly mouse and partly human) monoclonal antibody that binds with high affinity to tumour necrosis factor and thus neutralises its activity.
- It is given by intravenous infusion at a dose of 3 mg/kg body weight at 0, two, and six weeks and at eight weekly intervals thereafter.
- Methotrexate is coadministered weekly to inhibit the production of neutralising antibodies. About half of patients who receive infliximab develop new positive autoantibodies, but the development of lupus like syndrome is rare.
- Anaphylactic reactions have been reported, so it should only be administered in specialist units with adequate resuscitation facilities.

Adalimumab

- Adalimumab is a fully human monoclonal anti-tumour necrosis factor antibody.
- It has low immunogenicity and so does not need coadministration of methotrexate, although the combination is safe.
- It is administered by weekly or fortnightly subcutaneous injections.

Anakinra

- Anakinra is a recombinant human interleukin-1 receptor antagonist.
- It is administered by daily subcutaneous injections of 100 mg.
- Injection site reaction is seen commonly, but it rarely forces the cessation of therapy. Neutropenia is seen occasionally.

Diet and arthritis

For centuries sufferers from rheumatic disease have been advised to alter their diet in the hope of improving their disease. No evidence that this changes the natural history exists, but some symptomatic relief might be obtained. Whether the basis of diet therapy lies in supplements of trace elements or antioxidants or in avoiding "toxic" or "allergenic" constituents remains to be determined.

Evidence shows that starvation produces short-term improvements in the activity of rheumatoid arthritis. This raises the possibility that dietary manipulation has something to offer.

Whichever way diet modification is pursued, suspicious foodstuffs must be tested by repeated reintroduction, as extreme dietary exclusions may induce deficiency disorders.

Food supplements

A wide variety of supplements have been tried by patients suffering from rheumatoid arthritis. They may be introducing anti-inflammatory food additives. The benefits for rheumatoid arthritis are claimed rather than actually proven at present.

Dietary therapy
- Avoidance of foods thought to worsen synovitis:
  Dairy products
  Cereals
  Eggs
- Elimination diet
  Consists of "non-allergenic" foods such as rice, carrots, or fish followed by graded reintroduction

Food supplements
- Selenium supplementation
- Extract from New Zealand green lipped mussel
- Fish oil
- Evening primrose oil

Further reading

- van de Putte LB, van Gestel AM, van Riel PL. Early treatment of rheumatoid arthritis: rationale, evidence, and implications. *Ann Rheum Dis.*1998;57:511-12
- Geborek P, Crnkic M, Petersson IF, Saxne T. South Swedish Arthritis Treatment Group. Etanercept, infliximab, and leflunomide in established rheumatoid arthritis: clinical experience using a structured follow up programme in southern Sweden. *Ann Rheumatic Dis* 2002;61:793-8
- Weinblatt ME, Reda D, Henderson W, Giobbie-Hurder A, Williams D, Diani A, et al. Sulfasalazine treatment for rheumatoid arthritis: a meta-analysis of 15 randomized trials. *J Rheumatol* 1999;26:2123-30
- Capell HA, Porter DR, Madhok R, Hunter JA. Second line (disease modifying) treatment in rheumatoid arthritis: which drug for which patient? *Ann Rheum Dis* 1993;52:423-8
- Felson DT, Anderson JJ, Meenan RF. Use of short-term efficacy/toxicity tradeoffs to select second-line drugs in rheumatoid arthritis. *Arthritis Rheum* 1992;35:1117-25
- Felson DT, Anderson JJ, Meenan RF. The comparative efficacy and toxicity of second-line drugs in rheumatoid arthritis. *Arthritis Rheum* 1990;33:1449-61
- Jobanputra P, Barton P, Bryan S, Fry-Smith A, Burls A. The clinical effectiveness and cost-effectiveness of new drug treatments for rheumatoid arthritis: etanercept and infliximab. *NICE* 2001. www.nice.org.uk/pdf/RAAssessmentReport.pdf
- Emery P, Breedveld FC, Dougados M, Kalden JR, Schiff MH, Smolen JS. Early referral recommendation for newly diagnosed rheumatoid arthritis: evidence based development of a clinical guide. *Ann Rheum Dis* 2002;61:290-7
- Vries C de. Effects of TNF-alpha antagonists in people with rheumatoid arthritis. In: Foxcroft DR, Muthu V, eds. STEER: Succinct and Timely Evaluated Evidence Reviews 2002;2. Wessex Institute for Health Research and Development, University of Southampton. www.signpoststeer.org
- Vries C de. Cox-II inhibitors versus non-steroidal anti-inflammatory drugs in rheumatoid arthritis and osteoarthritis patients: gastrointestinal effects. In: Foxcroft DR, Muthu V, eds. STEER: Succinct and Timely Evaluated Evidence Reviews 2002;2. Wessex Institute for Health Research and Development, University of Southampton. www.signpoststeer.org
- Maetzel A, Wong A, Strand V, Tugwell P, Wells G, Bombardier C. Meta-analysis of treatment termination rates among rheumatoid arthritis patients receiving disease-modifying anti-rheumatic drugs. *Rheumatology* 2000;39:975-81
- Van den Ende CH, Vliet Vlieland TP, Munneke M, Hazes JM. Dynamic exercise therapy in rheumatoid arthritis: a systematic review. *Br J Rheumatol* 1998;37:677-87
- Muller H, de Toledo FW, Resch KL. Fasting followed by vegetarian diet in patients with rheumatoid arthritis: a systematic review. *Scand J Rheumatol* 2001;30:1-10
- Laine L, Bombardier C, Hawkey CJ, Davis B, Shapiro D, Brett C, et al. Stratifying the risk of NSAID-related upper gastrointestinal clinical events: results of a double-blind outcomes study in patients with rheumatoid arthritis. *Gastroenterology* 2002;23:1006-12
- Fortin PR, Lew RA, Liang MH, Wright EA, Beckett LA, Chalmers TC, et al. Validation of a meta-analysis: the effects of fish oil in rheumatoid arthritis. *J Clin Epidemiology* 1995;48:1379-90
- Volker D, Fitzgerald P, Major G, Garg M. Efficacy of fish oil concentrate in the treatment of rheumatoid arthritis. *J Rheumatology* 2000;27:2343-6
- Gøtzsche PC. Reporting of outcomes in arthritis trials measured on ordinal and interval scales is inadequate in relation to meta-analysis. *Ann Rheum Dis* 2001;60:349-52
- Pisetsky DS, St Clair EW. Progress in the treatment of rheumatoid arthritis. *JAMA* 2001;286:2787-90

13　Spondyloarthropathies

Gabrielle Kingsley, Non Pugh

What are spondyloarthropathies?

The spondyloarthropathies are a group of inflammatory arthritides involving the spine, sacroiliac joints, peripheral joints, and entheses. The group is linked by the association of spondyloarthropathies with the class I histocompatibility molecule human leucocyte antigen B27.

The 1991 criteria of the European Spondyloarthropathy Study Group are often used to define spondyloarthropathy. To fulfil them, patients must have inflammatory spinal pain, synovitis (asymmetrical/lower limb), or both, with one or more of alternating buttock pain, enthesopathy, sacroiliitis, family history, psoriasis, or inflammatory bowel disease.

Who gets spondyloarthropathies?

Spondyloarthropathies affect young adults and are more common in males. Their overall prevalence is 0.5-1%, with racial and geographical variation. They can be triggered by a variety of conditions, including non-specific urethritis, gastroenteritis, psoriasis, or inflammatory bowel disease.

What causes spondyloarthropathies?

Both genetic and environmental factors seem to be involved in the pathogenesis of spondyloarthropathies. Abnormalities in the bowel may also play a role.

Genetic factors

A significant role for genetic factors is suggested by strong family clustering and a twin concordance rate of 24-60%. Human leucocyte antigen B27 is the most important genetic risk factor, but its role in pathogenesis is unclear. Studies in West African, Sardinian, and Thai populations suggest certain human leucocyte antigen-B27 alleles may not be associated with disease, but these remain controversial. Additional susceptibility factors include genes for other class I and II major histocompatibility complex, genes for cytokines, and the gene for CYP2D6 (a cytochrome P450 enzyme).

Examples of spondyloarthropathies

- Ankylosing spondylitis
- Psoriatic arthritis (inflammatory arthritis associated with psoriasis)
- Reactive arthritis (arthritis following triggering enteric or genitourinary infection)
- Enteropathic arthritis (arthritis associated with inflammatory bowel disease)
- Undifferentiated spondyloarthropathy

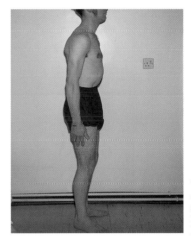

Typical "question mark" posture of a patient with long-standing spondylitis with loss of lumbar lordosis and exaggerated thoracic kyphosis

---

Prevalence of spondyloarthropathies

Spondyloarthropathy	Prevalence in United Kingdom	Sex ratio	HLAB27 +ve
Ankylosing spondylitis	150 per 100 000	4:1 (male to female)	90%
Psoriatic arthritis	100 per 100 000	1:1 (male to female)	
• Peripheral			20%
• Spinal			50%
Reactive arthritis	30 per 100 000	3:1 (male to female)	60-75%
Enteropathic arthritis	2-20% patients with inflammatory bowel disease		
• Peripheral		Female > male	No increase
• Spinal		Male > female	50%

Environmental factors

Infection is the other major aetiological factor. Reactive arthritis is triggered by gastroenteritis or urethritis and,

Studies show that reactive arthritis is caused by an immune response to bacterial antigens that have migrated from the primary site of infection to the joint

although triggering bacteria cannot be grown from the joint, bacterial antigen or DNA can be found by immunological or polymerase chain reaction techniques. In addition, anti-bacterial T cell responses can be found in the joint.

Another rare infection-related disease that is often classified as a spondyloarthropathy is Whipple's disease. It comprises peripheral arthritis (occasionally spondylitis or sacroiliitis), lymphadenopathy, abdominal pain, and diarrhoea, and it responds to antibiotic treatment. Pathologically, masses of infiltrating macrophages are found in the small intestine, lymph nodes, and synovium; these contain periodic acid Schiff positive material, identified as rod-shaped bacilli by electron microscopy. Recently, these organisms have been identified by polymerase chain reaction as a new Gram-positive actinomycete, *Tropheryma whippeli*, but the organism is difficult to culture.

No evidence shows that other spondyloarthropathies are caused by specific infections, although links between ankylosing spondylitis and *Klebsiella* and between psoriatic arthritis and streptococci have been proposed.

Bowel and spondyloarthropathies

The relation between inflammation in the bowel and spondyloarthropathy is evident from conditions like enteric reactive arthritis, Whipple's disease, and enteropathic arthritis. Studies with colonoscopies show bowel inflammation occurs in most spondyloarthropathies even without enteric symptoms; only a few of these patients subsequently progress to classical inflammatory bowel disease. Although the cause of the intestinal inflammation may vary, common factors include increased mucosal permeability (related to disease and non-steroidal anti-inflammatory drugs), persistent bacterial infection, and overgrowth of predominantly anaerobic bacteria. One hypothesis is that gut inflammation leads to enhanced mucosal permeability that allows bacteria or bacterial components (either from normal gut flora or pathogens) to pass across the gut wall and enter and activate macrophages. This leads to cytokine production and further inflammation, and the macrophages transport bacteria systemically to the lymphoid tissue and joints.

What should make you suspect a spondyloarthropathy?

Musculoskeletal features

Inflammatory back pain has two components: sacroiliitis and spondylitis. Sacroiliitis presents with bilateral, unilateral, or alternating buttock pain. Spondylitis manifests initially as low back pain, although it ultimately may affect any level from the neck to the sacrum. Spinal movements are usually restricted. Inflammatory back pain is worse after periods of inactivity and in the early morning (early morning stiffness). Severely affected patients may wake from sleep in the early hours of the morning and be unable to "lie in" at weekends. In contrast, the symptoms of mechanical back pain are worse with activity and toward the end of the day.

Enthesitis (inflammation of the entheses—the sites of insertion of ligaments and tendons into bone) manifests as local tenderness and pain after use of the relevant muscles. Common sites include the plantar fascia and the insertion of the Achilles tendon. These conditions can also arise because of mechanical stress but are more likely to be related to spondyloarthropathy if they are multiple and unresponsive to treatment.

Peripheral arthritis presents as pain and swelling in one or more joints. It usually is asymmetrical and it classically affects the lower limbs.

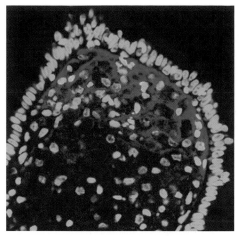

Fluorescent in situ hybridisation of a small intestinal biopsy in a case of Whipple's disease (confocal laser scanning microscopy). *Tropheryma whippeli* rRNA is blue, nuclei of human cells are green and the intracellular cytoskeletal protein vimentin red. Magnification about × 200

Characteristic clinical features of spondyloarthropathies in different systems

Musculoskeletal
- Sacroiliitis
- Spondylitis
- Enthesitis
- Peripheral arthritis

Eye
- Conjunctivitis
- Iritis

Gastrointestinal
- Inflammatory bowel disease
- Diarrhoea

Skin and nails
- Psoriasis
- Keratoderma blenorrhagica
- Nail disease

Genitourinary
- Urethritis
- Cervicitis

Cardiovascular (rare)
- Aortic regurgitation
- Cardiac conduction defects

Spondyloarthropathies usually occur in young patients (those aged 20-40 years) and are more common in men

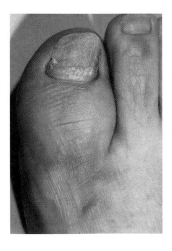

Dactylitis (sausage toe)—swelling of both joint and soft tissue is typical of spondyloarthropathy and contrasts with rheumatoid arthritis where swelling of joint alone leads to fusiform appearance

Skin and nails

All patients with suspected spondyloarthropathy should be carefully examined for psoriasis. As well as occurring in the common sites, such as the knees and elbows, psoriasis may occur in less obvious sites, including the scalp, natal cleft, umbilicus, genitalia, and feet.

Patients with reactive arthritis may have a psoriaform lesion that affects only the palms of the hands and the soles of the feet. This is known as keratoderma blenorrhagica.

Nail disease presents as onycholysis (separation of the nail bed from the nail) or nail pitting. It occurs commonly in psoriatic arthritis and rarely in reactive arthritis.

Eye

Iritis (anterior uveitis) occurs in 5% of patients with spondyloarthropathies. In some spondyloarthropathies, it is even more common: the lifetime risk in ankylosing spondylitis is 10-25%. All patients should be warned in advance about this complication and told that urgent ophthalmological review is needed if they develop an acute red eye.

Conjunctivitis is a characteristic feature of reactive arthritis (and occasionally other spondyloarthropathies). It presents with grittiness and soreness, rather than acute pain, in the eye. If any doubt exists as to whether the lesion could be iritis, however, the patient should be referred for an expert opinion.

Gut

Patients with enteropathic arthritis present with the full range of symptoms associated with inflammatory bowel disease (Crohn's or ulcerative colitis). Patients with enteric reactive arthritis may present with gastroenteritis. As discussed in the section on pathogenesis, changes suggestive of inflammatory bowel disease have been found in many patients with spondyloarthropathies. Some of these patients, on closer questioning, admit to low level diarrhoea, although many others are asymptomatic.

Genitourinary

Urethritis and cervicitis occur in reactive arthritis. In sexually acquired reactive arthritis, they occur after the triggering infection with *Chlamydia trachomatis*. They can also occur, however, in sexually acquired and enteric reactive arthritis, as non-infectious secondary disease manifestations. Circinate balanitis is another secondary manifestation of reactive arthritis.

What else might it be?

The differential diagnosis of spondyloarthropathy depends on the clinical features with which it presents.

What investigations should be done?

Haematology, biochemistry, immunology, and tissue typing

Full blood count may show anaemia caused by chronic disease or bleeding in patients who are on non-steroidal anti-inflammatory drugs. The acute phase response may be raised in patients with active disease, although this is less marked in patients without peripheral arthritis.

Biochemical tests should be performed in patients who have gastrointestinal symptoms or are on long-term therapy with non-steroidal anti-inflammatory drugs or antirheumatic drugs. Other blood tests, including rheumatoid factor, autoantibodies (which are negative in spondyloarthropathies),

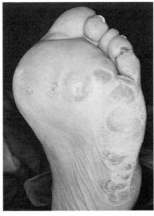
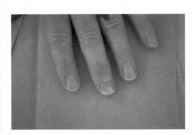

Left: keratoderma blenorrhagica—psoriaform lesion seen in reactive arthritis, which only affects the palms and soles. Right: psoriatic nail involvement (onycholysis) with asymmetrical distal and proximal interphalangeal arthritis

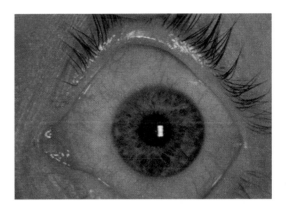

Conjuctivitis in a patient with reactive arthritis

Common differential diagnoses for spondyloarthropathy

Back or buttock pain
- Mechanical back pain
- Other causes of back pain (non-skeletal, infection, metabolic bone disease, and malignancy)

Enthesitis
- Mechanical soft tissue problems

Monoarthritis
- Septic arthritis
- Crystal arthritis
- Trauma, rarely osteoarthritis

Polyarthritis (rare)
- Rheumatoid arthritis
- Other chronic inflammatory arthropathies

Investigations most often used in diagnosis of spondyloarthropathies

Haematology
- Full blood count
- Acute phase response (erythrocyte sedimentation rate, C-reactive protein, and plasma viscosity)

Biochemistry
- Urea and electrolytes, liver and bone biochemistry, serum urate (in specific circumstances)

Immunology and tissue typing
- Rheumatoid factor and autoantibodies (for differential diagnosis)
- HLA B27 not generally useful

Microbiology
- Urethral or cervical swabs
- Stool cultures
- Antibacterial antibody titres not generally useful

Joint aspiration
- Microscopy of synovial fluid for microbes and crystals
- Synovial fluid culture

Imaging
- Radiography
- Radionuclide scan
- Computed tomography
- Magnetic resonance imaging

and serum urate may be needed to exclude specific differential diagnoses if the patient's clinical presentation suggests their presence.

Tissue typing for human leucocyte antigen B27 generally is not useful in diagnosis because of its low positive predictive value. This is because, although it is sensitive (in ankylosing spondylitis, 90% of those affected are positive), it is not specific (10% of normal Caucasian populations are positive), and spondyloarthropathies are much rarer than their common differential diagnoses such as mechanical back pain. Its use should be reserved for specialists.

Microbiology

Urethral or cervical swabs should be performed in any patient likely to have *Chlamydia trachomatis* non-specific urethritis; those in whom the diagnosis is strongly suspected should be referred to a specialist clinic for investigation. Stool cultures are valuable only in those with a positive history of diarrhoea. Antibacterial antibody tests are rarely of value and should not be performed routinely. This is because either good serological tests do not exist (for example, for *Shigella*) or exposure is so common that many people will be positive (for example, for *Chlamydia*).

Joint aspiration

In patients who present with monoarthritis, joint aspiration is needed to exclude septic or crystal arthritis. Joint fluid should be sent for microscopy and Gram staining (for bacteria), polarised light microscopy (for urate or pyrophosphate crystals), and culture. In immunosuppressed patients or those with chronic synovitis, infection with atypical organisms such as *Mycobacteria* or fungi should be considered. In the future, synovial fluid may be tested by polymerase chain reaction, not only for bacterial DNA associated with septic arthritis but also for chlamydial DNA associated with reactive arthritis.

Imaging

In ankylosing spondylitis, plain radiographs of the sacroiliac joints ultimately will show bilateral sacroiliitis, although changes may take up to two years to develop. Initially, erosions are seen on the iliac side, with apparent widening of the joint followed by sclerosis and ankylosis. In the lumbar spine, early radiographic changes include squaring of the vertebrae and bony bridging between the vertebrae (syndesmophytes). After several years of severe disease, complete fusion of the spine ("bamboo spine") may develop. Radiographs in chronic enthesitis may show erosions and bony spurs.

In psoriatic arthritis, spinal and sacroiliac radiographs are similar to those in patients with ankylosing spondylitis, but unilateral or asymmetrical sacroiliitis is more common, and syndesmophytes are thicker and more horizontal. Typical abnormalities of the peripheral joints include erosions, sclerosis of the joint margins, bony proliferation cysts, and ankylosis. More severe cases may show destruction of bone ends or the "pencil-in cup" deformity, in which the distal end of one phalanx impacts into the base of the next.

Radiographs are usually unhelpful in reactive and enteropathic arthritis, unless the condition is longstanding, in which case lesions similar to the above may be seen.

Quantified radionuclide scans of the sacroiliac joints can detect inflammatory changes as increased uptake. Scans from computed tomography (to detect early erosions) or magnetic resonance imaging (to detect sacroiliac joint inflammation or early erosion) are used increasingly as they seem to be more sensitive. These are useful particularly in the early stages of disease, when plain radiographs are unhelpful or equivocal.

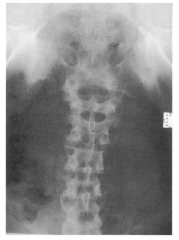

Radiograph of spine showing thoracolumbar syndesmophytes (longitudinal ligamentous calcifications)

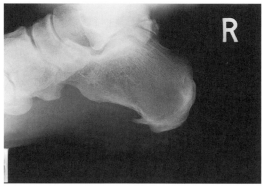

Radiograph showing early calcaneal spur on heel of patient with chronic plantar fasciitis, a common form of enthesitis

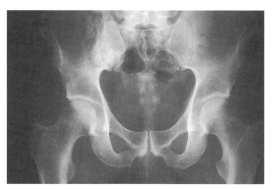

Sacroiliac joint radiograph in patient with psoriatic arthritis showing unilateral sacroiliitis

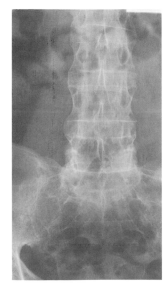

Lumbar spine radiograph in psoriatic arthritis with typical asymmetrical changes. On the left (patient's right) is extensive syndesmophyte formation, producing the classical "bamboo spine" appearance of spondylitis. On the right (patient's left) are early syndesmophytes. Courtesy of Professor Roger Sturrock, University of Glasgow

Individual spondyloarthropathies

Most patients with spondyloarthropathy have a defined disease: ankylosing spondylitis, psoriatic arthritis, reactive arthritis, or enteropathic arthritis. Some patients do not, however, fully fit the criteria for any of these. Such patients should be classified as having undifferentiated spondyloarthropathy, as long as they meet the 1991 criteria of the European Spondyloarthropathy Study Group. Their diagnosis should be reviewed regularly, as they often progress to a more classic spondyloarthropathy.

Moll and Wright classified psoriatic arthritis into five subsets (mono or oligoarthritis, distal interphalangeal joint arthritis, rheumatoid-like polyarthritis, spondylitis, and arthritis mutilans). Apart from arthritis mutilans, these subsets do not seem to be stable, as mono or oligoarthritis may evolve into polyarthritis and spondylitis occurs with any type.

The classic infections that trigger reactive arthritis include sexually-acquired reactive arthritis, *Chlamydia trachomatis* urethritis, and, for enteric reactive arthritis, gastroenteritis due to *Salmonella*, *Shigella*, *Yersinia*, or *Campylobacter*. *Streptococcus* causes a reactive polyarthritis not associated with human leucocyte antigen-B27. Cases of reactive arthritis associated with other bacteria have been described, but causation has not been proven.

Other enteric causes of arthritis or spondyloarthropathy include Whipple's disease, coeliac disease, and intestinal bypass surgery for obesity.

Psoriatic arthritis

Common presentations	• Psoriasis (may precede or follow onset of arthritis)
	• Monoarthritis or dactylitis (sausage fingers and/or toes)
Other locomotor features	• Oligoarthritis or polyarthritis
	• Inflammatory spinal pain
	• Enthesitis
Systemic features	• Nail changes in 80% compared to 20% of patients with uncomplicated psoriasis
	• Amyloidosis
Complications	• As for ankylosing spondylitis if spinal psoriatic arthritis
Natural history	• Recurrent or progressive usually non-erosive arthritis
	• Rapid progression to severe deformity rare except in arthritis mutilans subset where it is characteristic
	• Psoriasis and arthritis worse in HIV positive patients

Enteropathic arthritis

Common presentations	• Crohn's disease or ulcerative colitis
	• Lower limb peripheral arthritis
	• Inflammatory spinal pain
Other locomotor features	• Enthesitis
	• Tendonitis
Systemic features	• Features of inflammatory bowel disease
Complications	• As for ankylosing spondylitis if spinal disease plus complications of inflammatory bowel disease
Natural history	• Recurrent or progressive usually non-erosive arthritis

Ankylosing spondylitis

Common presentations	• Inflammatory low back and buttock pain
Other locomotor features	• Enthesitis
	• Peripheral arthritis (relatively rare)
Systemic features	• Iritis (10-25%)
	• Aortic regurgitation or cardiac conduction defects (rare)
	• Apical pulmonary fibrosis (rare)
Complications	• Chest infection caused by reduced expansion of chest wall
	• Fractures of rigid segments of spine, for example, neck
	• Cauda equina syndrome
	• Amyloidosis
	• Disease outcome variable
Natural history	• Inflammation can remit in later life but symptoms may persist because of secondary degenerative change
	• No increase in mortality but morbidity from systemic features and complications in severe cases

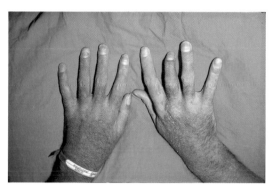

Hands in psoriatic arthritis showing asymmetrical polyarthropathy of the distal and proximal interphalangeal and metacarpophalangeal joints, with skin and nail changes

Reactive arthritis

Common presentations	• Non-specific urethritis/gastroenteritis followed after 1-4 weeks by lower limb mono/oligoarthritis or dactylitis
	• Triad of arthritis, conjunctivitis, and urethritis (previously known as Reiter's syndrome)
Other locomotor features	• Inflammatory spinal pain
	• Enthesitis
Systemic features	• Urethritis, cervicitis, and circinate balanitis
	• Conjunctivitis and rarely iritis
	• Keratoderma blenorrhagica and rarely nail changes
	• Carditis (very rare)
	• Amyloidosis
Complications	• As for ankylosing spondylitis if spinal psoriatic arthritis
	• Most first attacks resolve but can recur
Natural history	• Rarely progresses to chronic reactive arthritis or ankylosing spondylitis (more usual in sexually-acquired reactive arthritis)

Management of spondyloarthropathies

The management of a patient with a spondyloarthropathy depends on the specific diagnosis and on the particular clinical problems affecting the patient.

Non-drug therapy

Physiotherapy is a crucial part of the treatment of inflammatory spinal disease from its onset. All patients should be referred for formal assessment and treatment with a physiotherapist with expertise in this condition. Patients learn a daily exercise programme that relieves pain and stiffness and improves posture and spinal movement. Some patients will also need other physiotherapy treatments, such as hydrotherapy to improve mobility or ultrasound to treat enthesitis.

Surgery is used in the later stages of disease. The most usual intervention needed is total joint replacement for the hips (especially in ankylosing spondylitis), the knees, or, more rarely, the shoulders. Surgery also may be needed to treat some soft tissue problems or certain complications such as spinal fracture.

Drugs for symptom relief

Non-steroidal anti-inflammatory drugs usually provide more effective relief of pain and stiffness than simple analgesics, although analgesics may have a place in patients intolerant of non-steroidal anti-inflammatory drugs. Most patients should be treated with standard non-steroidal anti-inflammatory drugs but in those who are older or who have gastrointestinal symptoms, cyclooxygenase-2 inhibitors or prophylaxis with proton pump inhibitors should be considered.

Local steroid injections can be used for arthritis or enthesitis. Short courses of systemic corticosteroids may occasionally be considered for severe unresponsive peripheral joint symptoms, but they have little effect on the spine. They are best avoided in patients with psoriasis as they may exacerbate the skin disease.

Disease modifying antirheumatic drugs

Disease modifying antirheumatic drugs are used in patients with persistent peripheral arthritis especially if erosive or destructive changes are developing. The main drugs used are sulfasalazine and methotrexate (which can also treat skin psoriasis) and less commonly azathioprine. Though these drugs are standard treatments, the clinical trial evidence supporting their use is relatively limited, particularly with regard to altering bone erosion or disease outcome. These drugs also have little or no effect on spinal disease.

In contrast, anti-tumour necrosis factor α therapy has been shown, in controlled clinical trials, to improve peripheral and spinal disease in ankylosing spondylitis and psoriatic arthritis. The monoclonal antibody infliximab, which is given six weekly by infusion, and the soluble receptor etanercept, which is given twice weekly by subcutaneous injection, have been shown to be effective, although as yet they are licensed only for rheumatoid arthritis and juvenile idiopathic arthritis. Further anti-tumour necrosis factor α agents are in development. These agents are likely to prove to be important treatments for patients with severe disease, particularly spinal disease that is unresponsive to other therapy. The cost and significant side effect profile (especially infection) are likely to preclude their use in patients with milder disease.

Treatments for spondyloarthropathy

Non-drug treatments	• Physiotherapy
	• Surgery
Drugs to relieve symptoms	• Non-steroidal anti-inflammatory drugs
	• Local corticosteroid injections
	• Systemic corticosteroids (rare)
Disease modifying antirheumatic drugs	• Sulfasalazine
	• Methotrexate
	• Azathioprine
Drugs to prevent disease	• Anti-tumour necrosis factor alpha therapy
	• Antibiotics

Further reading

General

- Calin A, Taurog JD, eds. *The spondylarthritides.* Oxford: Oxford University Press, 1998

Pathogenesis

- Brown MA, Crane AM, Wordsworth BPW. Genetic aspects of susceptibility, severity and clinical expression in ankylosing spondylitis. *Curr Op Rheumatol* 2002;14:354-60
- Kingsley G. Infection in the pathogenesis of rheumatoid arthritis. In: Firestein GS, Panayi GS, Wollheim FA, eds. *Rheumatoid Arthritis: Frontiers in pathogenesis and treatment.* Oxford: Oxford University Press, 2000
- Kingsley G. Microbial DNA in the synovium—a role in aetiology or a mere bystander? *Lancet* 1997;349:1038-9
- Baeten D, De Keyser F, Mielants H, Veys EM. Immune linkages between inflammatory bowel disease and spondyloarthropathies. *Curr Op Rheumatol* 2002;14:342-7

Clinical diseases

- Khan MA. Spondyloarthropathies: Editorial review. *Curr Op Rheumatol* 1997;9:281-3
- Gladman DD. Current concepts in psoriatic arthritis. *Curr Op Rheumatol* 2002;14:361-6
- Inman RD, Whittum-Hudson JA, Schumacher HR, Hudson AP. Chlamydia and associated arthritis. *Curr Op Rheumatol* 2000;12:254-62
- Toivanen A, Toivanen P. Reactive arthritis. *Curr Op Rheumatol* 2000;12:300-5
- Wollheim FA. Enteropathic arthritis: how do the joints talk with the gut? *Curr Op Rheumatol* 2001;13:305-9

Treatment

- Mease PJ, Goffe BS, Metz J, VanderStoep A, Finck B, Burge DJ. Etanercept in the treatment of psoriatic arthritis and psoriasis: a randomised trial. *Lancet* 2000;356:385-90
- Braun J, De Keyser F, Brandt J, Mielants H, Sieper J, Veys E. New treatment options in spondyloarthropathies: increasing evidence for significant efficacy of anti-tumor necrosis factor therapy. *Curr Op Rheumatol* 2001;13:245-50
- Braun J, Brandt J, Listing J, Zink A, Alten R, Golder W, et al. Treatment of active ankylosing spondylitis with infliximab: a randomised controlled multicentre trial. *Lancet* 2002;359:1187-93
- Braun J, Sieper J. Therapy of ankylosing spondylitis and other spondyloarthritides: established medical treatment, anti-TNF-alpha therapy and other novel approaches. *Arthritis Res.* 2002;4:307-21

Disease prevention

Antibiotic treatment, usually with tetracyclines, is indicated for non-specific urethritis, as it prevents progression to reactive arthritis, as well as pelvic inflammatory disease. Gastroenteritis, in this as in other situations, should not be treated with antibiotics. Despite some early suggestions of benefit, studies using a variety of antibiotics have shown that these drugs overall have no convincing effect on the duration or severity of arthritis in sexually-acquired or enteric reactive arthritis.

14 Juvenile idiopathic arthritis

Mark Friswell, Tauny R Southwood

The diagnosis of arthritis and other rheumatic diseases in children needs an awareness of the conditions, well honed clinical skills, and the patience to complete a meticulous physical examination of a potentially fractious child. It can be all too easy to dismiss the relatively common paediatric symptoms of fever, rash, listlessness, weakness, anorexia, or pain as secondary to insignificant viral illnesses, which leads to delay in diagnosis and the start of appropriate treatment. The overzealous investigator may raise anxiety levels in the child and parents, however, perpetuating or even exacerbating non-organic debility. This chapter aims to give an overview of juvenile idiopathic arthritis and its clinical features, differential diagnosis, investigations, natural history, and principles of treatment. No substitute exists, however, for actual clinical experience, and you are strongly recommended to practise the skills of paediatric musculoskeletal examination at every appropriate opportunity. An appreciation of normality is an absolute prerequisite to the detection of abnormality.

Juvenile idiopathic arthritis is the umbrella term that encompasses previous nomenclature including Still's disease, juvenile rheumatoid arthritis, or juvenile chronic arthritis. The hallmark for diagnosis in a child is persistent joint swelling in the absence of any defined cause. At least seven different forms of the disease exist. In total, 95% of patients with juvenile idiopathic arthritis have a disease that is clinically and immunogenetically distinct from rheumatoid arthritis in adults.

Clinical features

Juvenile idiopathic arthritis is one of the most common physically disabling conditions of childhood, with a prevalence of about one in a thousand children under the age of 16 years; that amounts to over 12 000 affected children in the United Kingdom. The incidence of juvenile idiopathic arthritis, however, is only one in 10 000. In a typical general practice, a general practitioner is likely to see only one new case every 20 years. It is difficult to maintain a high index of suspicion for the diagnosis of juvenile idiopathic arthritis in the face of this degree of rarity.

History

Most affected children are in their preschool or early school years, and they often have difficulty describing such symptoms. Parents are likely to have noted joint swelling if one or more large peripheral joints are involved, such as the knee (the most common form of presentation), ankle, or wrist. Although it is rarer for children to present with isolated small joint (finger or toe) disease or axial joint involvement (such as the shoulder, hip, spine, or temporomandibular joints), parents are also less likely to have noted swelling in these joints, which potentially compounds the delay in diagnosis.

Physical signs

Peripheral joint arthritis in children is almost always accompanied by clinically detectable joint swelling. In the knee, this is usually demonstrable by a positive patella tap, ballottable

Key points

- Juvenile idiopathic arthritis is not the same disease as rheumatoid arthritis
- Juvenile idiopathic arthritis is characterised by persistent joint swelling
- Discomfort is common in juvenile idiopathic arthritis, pain less so
- Early diagnosis affects prognosis
- Aggressive treatment affects prognosis

Diagnosis of juvenile idiopathic arthritis

All three conditions must be met:
- Arthritis persisting for >6 weeks
- Onset before age 16
- Exclusion of other diseases causing arthritis

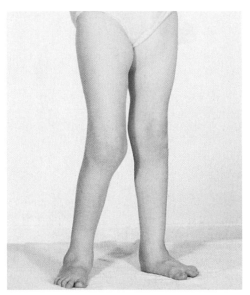

Oligoarthritis in a 3 year old girl

Typical symptoms of juvenile idiopathic arthritis

Constitutional	Localised to sites of pathology
• Fever	• Limping
• Rash	• Joint pain
• Tiredness	• Restricted joint movement
• Growth failure and visceral pain	• Joint swelling

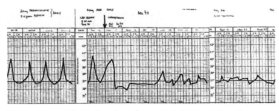

Temperature chart showing characteristic quotidian fever associated with systemic arthritis

synovial fluid, a palpable fluid thrill in the knee on flexing the joint, or occasionally a Baker's cyst in the popliteal fossa. Swelling of the ankle often obscures anterior tendon contours when the joint is dorsiflexed, although this may be difficult to see in chubby children. Wrist arthritis may be best appreciated by asking the child to press the palms of their hands together in the "prayer" position, when a dorsal bulge and reduced range of movement usually highlights the synovitis—especially if it is asymmetrical. Swelling of the elbow can be palpated on either side of the olecranon and usually results in a flexion deformity of the arm.

The small joints of the hands and feet should be inspected and palpated individually; usually reliable signs of synovitis are the presence of joint margin tenderness and restricted movement. Cervical spine involvement usually can be detected by inability to rotate the head laterally to place the chin on each shoulder and by reduced neck extension. Temporomandibular synovitis is often missed, but it usually prevents full and symmetrical opening of the mouth.

Once the presence of arthritis is confirmed objectively, it is vital to exclude conditions that may mimic juvenile idiopathic arthritis. Most serious among these are infection related (septic arthritis and reactive arthritis), trauma (including non-accidental injury), and neoplasia (such as acute lymphoblastic leukaemia and neuroblastoma).

Typical erythematosus evanescent rash of systemic arthritis. Often the rash is obvious only at the height of the fever and sometimes is confined to the axillary region and anterior chest wall

Differential diagnosis

Many diseases in childhood can present with joint or musculoskeletal symptoms. In broad terms they fall into one of four groups: mechanical disorders, inflammatory disorders, neoplasia, and the idiopathic pain syndromes.

Mechanical disorders
Joint pain secondary to hypermobility is the most common non-inflammatory diagnosis in patients newly referred to a paediatric rheumatology clinical service. A normal range of joint flexibility, which varies with age, sex, and ethnic background, is seen in childhood. In general, younger children are more flexible than older adolescents (babies and toddlers' joints are extremely mobile and the finding of flat feet in children of this age is normal), girls are more flexible than boys, and black children are more flexible than white. Much of the musculoskeletal pain is confined to the lower limbs and back. Lower limb findings may be improved by the use of custom moulded hard insoles (as indeed may other postural abnormalities of the feet) that aim to support the longitudinal foot arch and stabilise the ankle. To be successful, such insoles need specialised assessment and fitting. Most mechanical causes of joint pain tend to be worse after exercise and as the day goes on, but early morning stiffness the day or two after exercise may be a feature. Diffuse idiopathic musculoskeletal pain syndromes, such as fibromyalgia, have also been associated with hypermobility in school children.

Inflammatory disorders
Reactive arthritis—This is the most common form of arthritis in childhood. It is characterised by transient, painful, joint swelling (usually lasting less than six weeks), that follows, or rarely accompanies, evidence of extra-articular infection.

Septic arthritis—Almost exclusively monoarticular and associated with "pseudoparalysis" of the affected limb (extreme pain with the affected joint held rigidly in the position of maximum comfort). The child is usually systemically unwell, with a high fever and signs of toxicity. It is important, however,

Four groups of disorders cause joint musculoskeletal symptoms

- Mechanical disorders
- Inflammatory disorders
- Neoplasia
- Idiopathic pain syndromes

Common lower limb findings in hypermobility

- Pes planus
- Out-toeing gait
- Overpronated feet (secondary to ankle hypermobility)
- Genu recurvatum

Infective agents implicated in reactive arthritis

- Enteric bacteria are implicated in many paediatric cases of reactive arthritis
- Almost any infectious agent, including viruses (influenza, herpes, coxsackie, parvovirus B19, and rubella) and other bacteria, including mycoplasma, can be implicated
- Rheumatic fever and post-streptococcal reactive arthritis are both rare in European children, but they frequently occur in other parts of the world

to maintain a high index of suspicion of this condition in a child who is being, or has recently been, treated with antibiotics, because of the possibility of partially treated septic arthritis. Tuberculous septic arthritis may also present more insidiously. Blood cultures and joint aspiration for bacterial diagnosis should be undertaken before antibiotics are started. Arthrocentesis has the added advantage, particularly in the hip, of reducing intra-articular pressure and minimising the risk of compromised blood supply to the epiphysis. Intravenous antibiotics are usually advocated until 48 hours after defervescence, with oral antibiotics continued until the erythrocyte sedimentation rate has normalised and all clinical signs have settled.

Osteomyelitis—Particularly if located near a joint, this may cause a sterile effusion within that joint that may be mistaken for arthritis. X ray radiographs may be normal initially, so a technetium bone scan may be helpful to rule this out.

Systemic lupus erythematosus—This is rare in children and may have protean initial manifestations of which arthritis is but one. It typically presents in an adolescent girl with malaise, irritability, joint pain, and sometimes weight loss. An erythematous, acneiform facial rash may be present, but the classic photosensitive malar rash is found in less than one third of children with systemic lupus erythematosus. Tests for antinuclear antibodies are almost always positive, but more specific antibodies such as those to double-stranded DNA and Sm are less frequent in childhood. Lymphopaenia, thrombocytopaenia, and evidence of complement consumption are regular findings. Renal manifestations are the major cause of long-term morbidity and are more frequent in childhood than adult forms of systemic lupus erythematosus.

Juvenile dermatomyositis—This usually begins insidiously with malaise, progressive weakness (which may be mistaken for laziness) and erythematous facial rash (particularly around the eyes). Muscle pain is a common, if non-specific, symptom and arthritis is found in 30% of cases. The diagnosis of juvenile dermatomyositis is usually made on the basis of finding a symmetrical proximal myopathy, typical dermatological manifestations including Gottron's papules, and elevated serum muscle enzymes. Respiratory failure and aspiration pneumonia may be life threatening.

Henoch-Schönlein purpura—The most common vasculitis of childhood, this presents with a purpuric rash over the lower legs and buttocks, which usually is associated with arthritis of the ankles or knees and occasionally abdominal pain. Haematuria and proteinuria may be found, but it is rare for significant renal disease to develop. Arthritis is an uncommon feature at presentation of other childhood vasculitides such as Kawasaki disease.

Neoplasia

Acute lymphoblastic leukaemia—may present with bone pain in children (sometimes primarily at night) and even frank arthritis, which can affect one or sometimes more joints.

Neuroblastoma—a particularly concerning possibility in younger children who present with features of systemic arthritis, metastasises early to bone, and causes pain that may be difficult for the doctor to localise.

Lymphoma—usually affects older children and may present with musculoskeletal symptoms.

Primary bone malignancies—rare and are usually visible on plain x ray radiographs.

Pain syndromes

The most dramatic musculoskeletal pain in children is often found in the idiopathic pain syndromes. These may be localised

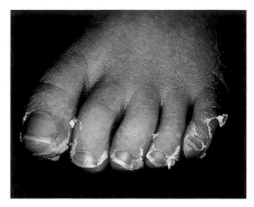
Localised scleroderma of the foot of an 11 year old girl

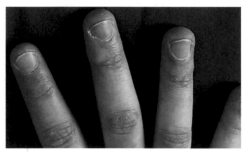
Gottron's papules in boy with juvenile dermatomyositis

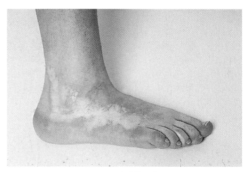
Desquamation of toes of child with Kawasaki disease

Benign tumours, such as osteoid osteoma, may present with night pain in a limb. They should be considered in the assessment of a child with "growing pains"

Features of complex regional pain syndrome

Characteristic	Occasional
• Severe pain	• Limb swelling
• Hyperaesthesia	• Mottling of skin
• Allodynia	• Cool pallor of skin
• Immobility of affected limb, even to extent of adopting bizarre posture	

(complex regional pain syndromes) or generalised (such as fibromyalgia). Exogenous stress (including school pressures, bullying or other forms of abuse, and even parental pressure) is a common accompanying feature, although often unrecognised by the parents. All such patients deserve meticulous physical examination and judicious investigation to rule out an underlying organic pathology. Overinvestigation and vacillating doctor-to-patient communication, however, may perpetuate or exacerbate the clinical features of these diseases. Occasionally, an idiopathic pain syndrome may complicate a pre-existing organic disease such as juvenile idiopathic arthritis. An individualised, intensive, multi-professional, rehabilitation regime, either in the community or inpatient based, is essential to restore function.

Complex regional pain syndromes—such as reflex sympathetic dystrophy, may begin after trauma (often minor) or without a clear precipitant.

Diffuse musculoskeletal pain syndromes—characterised by disturbed sleep patterns (initial insomnia, exhausted awakening, and napping during day), tenderness over soft tissue "trigger" points (with facial grimacing and a sharp intake of breath), and the absence of other findings to suggest organic disease.

Investigations

The diagnosis of juvenile idiopathic arthritis is made on clinical features alone, as no pathognomonic investigations exist. Investigations are thus aimed at excluding a wide range of differential diagnoses.

Classification

Oligoarthritis: persistent
The most common form of juvenile idiopathic arthritis, oligoarthritis accounts for over half of all cases. It mainly affects preschool girls, with a sex ratio of 5 : 1. It is frequently associated with positive antinuclear antibodies. This group is thought to be at highest risk for the development of chronic anterior uveitis (20%). Chronic anterior uveitis is clinically silent and insidiously progressive; it produces visual loss and even blindness if not detected by slit lamp examination and treated early.

Extended oligoarthritis
One third of children whose disease begins with an oligoarticular pattern during the first six months of the disease will continue to develop arthritis in further joints thereafter, hence the nomenclature "extended." These patients have a different immunogenetic background to patients with persistent oligoarthritis. They seem to have a poorer prognosis and still have the same frequency of chronic anterior uveitis as patients who remain oligoarticular.

Psoriatic juvenile idiopathic arthritis
Arthritis may predate the onset of the classical skin findings of psoriasis by many years. The pattern of articular involvement in psoriatic arthritis is often asymmetrical, and it affects both small and large joints in a similar way to extended oligoarthritis, except for the characteristic extra-articular features of psoriasis.

Enthesitis related arthritis
This form of juvenile idiopathic arthritis is likely to be the precursor illness to ankylosing spondylitis during the adult years. It typically begins after the age of six years and affects

---

European League Against Rheumatism's classification of juvenile idiopathic arthritis
- Systemic onset
- Persistent oligoarticular
- Extended oligoarticular
- Polyarticular (rheumatoid factor negative)
- Polyarticular (rheumatoid factor positive)
- Psoriatic juvenile onset arthritis
- Enthesitis related arthritis

Investigations in children with arthritis

Radiology
- Plain x ray radiographs—to rule out fractures, avascular necrosis, bone neoplasia, bone dysplasia, osteomyelitis
- Ultrasonography—to confirm presence of joint effusion or to look for neuroblastoma
- Tech-99 bone scan—highlights bony inflammation secondary to infection, malignancy, or benign tumours such as osteoid osteoma

Haematology
- Full blood count—to exclude leukaemia
- Erythrocyte sedimentation rate—normal in up to half of patients with juvenile idiopathic arthritis
- Bone marrow aspirate—to exclude malignancy

Biochemistry
- C reactive protein—normal in up to half of patients with juvenile idiopathic arthritis
- Urinary catecholamines—to exclude neuroblastoma

Immunology
- Antinuclear antibodies—positive in only half of children with juvenile idiopathic arthritis and up to 5% of the general paediatric population.
- Rheumatoid factor—negative in 95% of children with juvenile idiopathic arthritis
- Immunoglobulins—to rule out immunoglobulin A-associated arthritis
- Antistreptolysin "O" titre and viral serology
- Borrelia Burgdorferi serology/polymerase chain reaction if history of travel in endemic areas

Synovial fluid analysis
- Mandatory in suspected septic arthritis, but does not help in other differential diagnoses

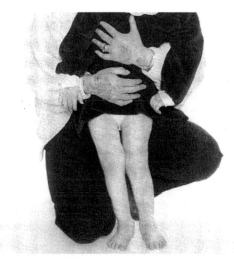

Psoriatic arthritis

boys more often than girls. It is characterised initially by lower limb arthritis and often is associated with enthesitis (inflammation of the point where tendon, ligament, or fascia inserts into bone). The most common enthesitic points are at the insertions of plantar fascia (calcaneum, the base of the fifth metatarsal, and the metatarsal heads), the insertion of the tendo Achillis into the calcaneum, and the enthesitic points around the patella. Symptoms of sacroiliitis and spinal arthritis are uncommon at presentation.

Polyarthritis: negative for rheumatoid factor

Polyarthritis accounts for 25-30% of patients, usually preschool girls with a predominantly symmetrical arthritis that affects upper and lower limbs. Chronic anterior uveitis and growth disturbance are important potential complications.

Polyarthritis: positive for rheumatoid factor

This form of juvenile idiopathic arthritis is similar in features and prognosis to adult rheumatoid arthritis. It presents in late childhood or adolescence and can be rapidly erosive. It affects 5% of patients with juvenile idiopathic arthritis.

Systemic arthritis

Systemic arthritis usually begins in early childhood (although it can occur at any age through to adulthood), with prominent extra-articular features. The systemic features usually resolve after the first few weeks. The pattern of arthritis is variable, ranging from oligoarthritis to a widespread polyarthritis that can be very difficult to control, and these children have the worst prognosis of all forms of juvenile idiopathic arthritis.

Treatment

The aim of therapy is to maintain the patient's quality of life and to preserve joint function for as long as the disease is active. Patient education and the support of an experienced paediatric rheumatology team are vital. The team should include a paediatric rheumatologist, and staff with specific paediatric expertise in rehabilitation, disease education, clinical and drug monitoring, school liaison, nutrition, family and social support, and psychology. In addition, ready access to other paediatric specialities—ophthalmology, orthopaedics, maxillofacial surgery, psychiatry, nephrology, and dermatology—is often needed.

Hospital admission should be considered for efficient initial investigation and team assessment of all patients with newly diagnosed acute arthritis, particularly if they are significantly disabled or have prominent systemic features. Most patients with juvenile idiopathic arthritis are managed in the outpatient setting, often as part of a clinical network that involves a paediatric rheumatology team in a tertiary referral centre together with a local team.

Drug treatment of juvenile idiopathic arthritis usually includes non-steroidal anti-inflammatory drugs and many patients need treatment with slow acting antirheumatic drugs such as methotrexate or sulfasalazine. Treatment with biological agents, including anti-tumour necrosis factor α preparations, are becoming more frequent. Repeat hospital admissions may be needed for intra-articular therapy and periods of intensive rehabilitation. As with all chronic treatment, the issue of compliance is of particular importance in children. Drugs that need to be given more than twice daily should be avoided if possible, unpleasant tasting drugs are unlikely to be well tolerated, and other adverse effects undoubtedly reduce adherence to treatment, particularly in adolescence.

Extra-articular features of systemic arthritis

- Characteristic daily fever
- Evanescent erythematous macular rash
- Hepatomegaly
- Splenomegaly
- Lymphadenopathy
- Serositis

Members of local management team

- Paediatrician
- Rheumatologist
- Community paediatrician
- Community rehabilitation and support staff
- Patient's general practitioner

Differential diagnosis of juvenile idiopathic arthritis

Presenting with a single inflamed joint
- Juvenile idiopathic arthritis: oligoarticular, psoriatic, or enthesitis related
- Septic arthritis: bacterial or tubercular
- Lyme disease
- Reactive arthritis: secondary to bacterial or viral infections
- Haemarthrosis: secondary to trauma (including non-accidental) or bleeding disorder
- Malignancy: leukaemia or neuroblastoma most common

Presenting with more than one inflamed joint
- Juvenile idiopathic arthritis: polyarticular (positive or negative for rheumatoid factor), psoriatic, enthesitis related, or systemic onset
- Other connective tissue disease: systemic lupus erythematosus, juvenile dermatomyositis, sarcoidosis, Sjögren's syndrome, mixed connective tissue disease
- Reactive arthritis: secondary to bacterial or viral infections
- Lyme disease
- Malignancy: leukaemia or neuroblastoma most common
- Immunodeficiency associated arthritis
- Inflammatory bowel disease associated arthritis
- Other: chronic recurrent multifocal osteomyelitis, chronic infantile neurological cutaneous and arthritis syndrome, and periodic fevers

Presenting with systemic disease
- Systemic onset juvenile idiopathic arthritis
- Other connective tissue diseases—systemic lupus erythematosus, juvenile dermatomyositis, polyarteritis nodosa
- Infection: bacterial (streptococcal, including rheumatic fever, tuberculosis, *Gonococcus*, Lyme disease, and Brucella), viral (Epstein Barr virus and Hepatitis B), or parasitic (malaria)
- Inflammatory bowel disease
- Periodic fevers
- Chronic infantile neurological cutaneous and arthritis syndrome (CINCA—also known as NOMID: Neonatal-Onset Multisystem Inflammatory Disease)

Non-steroidal anti-inflammatory drugs

All children with active arthritis should receive regular non-steroidal anti-inflammatory drugs. These are used in higher doses, relative to body weight, than adults because children have increased rates of metabolism and renal excretion. An individual non-steroidal anti-inflammatory drug, if free of significant adverse effects, should be continued for 2-3 months before a judgment about efficacy is made. Cessation of non-steroidal anti-inflammatory drugs may be considered if the patient has been free of active disease for at least six months. Adverse effects include abdominal pain (usually minimised by taking the non-steroidal anti-inflammatory drug with food and treated successfully with ranitidine, omeprazole, or misoprostol), change in mood (usually transient), and rarely bronchospasm (but mild asthma does not seem to be a contraindication to the use of non-steroidal anti-inflammatory drugs in children).

Corticosteroids

Intra-articular preparations are the most frequently used form of corticosteroids in juvenile idiopathic arthritis. Triamcinolone hexacetonide has the highest efficacy and longest duration of action, although drug supplies are limited within the United Kindgom at present. Intra-articular medication in children is usually given under general anaesthesia, but the injection of one or two joints under local anaesthetic may be acceptable to older children.

Systemic steroids should be avoided if possible, because of the wide range of adverse effects, including growth suppression, in children. In some situations, however, intravenous methylprednisolone may help gain control of active polyarthritis, and it may even be lifesaving in the face of significant systemic arthritis with pericarditis. The use of oral prednisolone is limited to low dose, preferably alternate day, administration for children with severe polyarthritis.

Methotrexate

Methotrexate is effective in approximately 70% of children with polyarthritis but fewer with systemic disease. It should be considered for any child whose arthritis is not well controlled on non-steroidal anti-inflammatory drugs and intra-articular steroids alone. Initial doses of 0.3-0.5 mg/kg are usually given by mouth once a week and one hour before food to improve absorption. Doses are increased on a monthly basis if the arthritis is still uncontrolled, up to a maximum dose of 1 mg/kg/week. For recalcitrant disease, subcutaneous methotrexate provides serum levels up to 40% higher than the oral route.

Sulfasalazine

Sulfasalazine has been shown to be efficacious in oligoarthritis and polyarthritis, but seems particularly effective in enthesitis-related arthritis. Relatively high frequencies of dermatological adverse events and regimens of 2-4 doses per day have limited its use in juvenile idiopathic arthritis. It is of limited value in systemic onset juvenile idiopathic arthritis, with a poor clinical response and an increased incidence of side effects such as serum sickness, severe myelosuppression, and hepatitis.[1,2]

Anti-tumour necrosis factor α

Therapy with anti-tumour necrosis factor α has recently been advocated for the treatment of children with juvenile idiopathic arthritis whose disease is not adequately controlled on methotrexate or who are intolerant of it. Two drugs are currently available: etanercept and infliximab. There remain significant

---

Drug treatment

Non-steroidal anti-inflammatory drugs
- Ibuprofen 10 mg/kg/dose four times a day
- Piroxicam 0.2-0.3 mg/kg/dose once a day
- Naproxen 10 mg/kg/dose twice a day

Intra-articular steroids
Triamcinolone hexacetonide
- 1 mg/kg/joint for large joints
- 0.5 mg/kg/joint for medium joints
- 1-2.5 mg/joint for digits

Triamcinolone acetonide
- 2 mg/kg/joint for large joints
- 1 mg/kg/joint for medium joints
- 2-4 mg/joint for digits

Methotrexate*
- 0.3-1 mg/kg/dose once weekly oral or subcutaneously

Sulfasalazine*
- 25 mg/kg/dose twice daily

Etanercept*
- 0.4 mg/kg/dose twice weekly subcutaneously

Parenteral steroids
- Methylprednisolone 10-30 mg/kg/dose daily over 1-3 days
- Prednisolone 0.2-2 mg/kg/dose once a day

*Need regular monitoring with blood tests

The most common adverse event when using methotrexate is nausea, which is usually dose related, although paradoxically subcutaneous administration may be less of a problem in this regard than oral administration. Oral folate supplements or ondansetron may be helpful, as may psychologist support. Other side effects include abdominal pain; elevated liver enzymes; and rarely mouth ulcers, increased hair fall, and bone marrow suppression. Patients on methotrexate must have blood monitoring on a monthly basis to screen for abnormal liver function and bone marrow suppression

---

Anti-tumour necrosis factor α drugs
Etanercept
- Given by subcutaneous injection twice weekly
- Shown to be effective in over 80% of patients with juvenile idiopathic arthritis previously treated with methotrexate, with relatively few short-term adverse effects

Infliximab
- Given by intravenous infusion every six weeks

long-term concerns relating to the potential disruption of immune surveillance in this class of biologic agents.

Other drug medication

Hydroxychloroquine—has been used widely for adjunctive therapy of polyarthritis in the past, but it has largely been superseded by other medication.

Cyclophosphamide—used occasionally for patients unresponsive to the above therapies, particularly in severe recalcitrant systemic arthritis.

Autologous stem cell bone marrow transplantation—being investigated for juvenile idiopathic arthritis unresponsive to all other therapy. It is a high risk procedure but seems to offer a reasonable chance of inducing disease remission.

Natural history

Juvenile idiopathic arthritis may remit spontaneously, but objective predictors of this outcome are lacking. Long-term follow up studies have highlighted a rather poorer prognosis for juvenile idiopathic arthritis than previously believed. Anecdotal evidence shows that early diagnosis and rapid referral to an experienced paediatric rheumatology team is associated with improved outcome.

As many as 30% of children with juvenile idiopathic arthritis will continue to have active arthritis into their adult years, and many more will be left with the chronic sequelae of restricted joint movement, asymmetrical growth, and extra-articular abnormalities. An appreciation of this prognosis has imparted more urgency to starting aggressive treatment regimens than previously advocated

1 Brooks CD. Sulfasalazine for the management of juvenile rheumatoid arthritis. *J Rheumatol* 2001;28:845-53
2 Jung JH, Jun JB, Yoo DH, Kim TH, Jung SS, Lee IH, et al. High toxicity of sulfasalazine in adult-onset Still's disease. *Clin Exp Rheumatol* 2000;18:245-8

15 Polymyalgia rheumatica and giant cell arteritis

Maya H Buch, Howard A Bird

Polymyalgia rheumatica is a clinical syndrome that affects older patients and comprises proximal muscle group stiffness, particularly in the shoulder, and systemic features such as fatigue and weight loss. It is associated with an increased erythrocyte sedimentation rate and responds dramatically to relatively small doses of steroids.

Giant cell arteritis is a systemic vasculitis that affects large and medium sized arteries. Although it may involve any artery, it has a propensity to affect the branches of the external carotid artery—particularly the posterior ciliary arteries that supply the optic nerve and the superficial temporal artery, hence its alternative (often interchangeable) name "temporal arteritis."

Increasingly it has become apparent that there is an overlap between temporal arteritis, giant cell arteritis, and polymyalgia rheumatica, and this leads to the concept that they are manifestations of a disease spectrum that affects the same disease population. The two entities may occur in the same patient simultaneously, at different time points, or independently. In giant cell arteritis, polymyalgia rheumatica has been observed in up to 60% of cases and vice versa in up to 80% of cases.

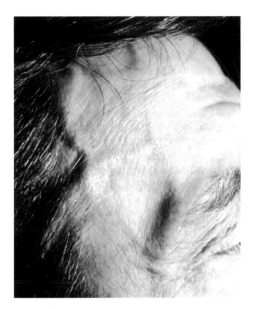

Giant cell arteritis. Involvement of the temporal artery is clearly seen

Causes

The cause of giant cell arteritis or polymyalgia rheumatica is likely to be polygenic, with both genetic and environmental factors contributing to disease susceptibility and severity.

Environmental
Acute onset prodromal events and synchronous variations in incidence of polymyalgia rheumatica and giant cell arteritis suggest a possible environmental infectious trigger. Several studies have shown concurrence in the incidence of polymyalgia rheumatica and giant cell arteritis with epidemics of *Mycoplasma pneumoniae*, *Chlamydia pneumoniae*, *Parvovirus B19*, *respiratory syncytial virus*, and *Adenovirus*. Despite this, no definite infectious agent has been identified.

Genetics
Racial differences in incidence and familial aggregation suggest a genetic susceptibility factor. Polymyalgia rheumatica and giant cell arteritis are linked with human leucocyte antigen-DR4. Patients that are DR4-positive and DR4-negative do not present differently. A conserved sequence within the second hypervariable region located in the antigen binding groove of the human leucocyte antigen-DR molecule has been identified.

Clinical features

In the absence of a diagnostic test, apart from biopsy of the temporal artery when giant cell arteritis is also present, diagnosis is based on clinical features and made by exclusion. Several diagnostic criteria sets have been suggested.

Epidemiology of polymyalgia rheumatica and giant cell arteritis

- Giant cell arteritis is the most common of the vasculitides, and polymyalgia rheumatica is more common than giant cell arteritis
- Pre-eminently affect Northern European subjects; can occur in any ethnic group
- Rare under age of 50 years
- Woman : man ratio = 3 : 1
- Annual incidence approximately 18 per 100 000 for giant cell arteritis and 100 per 100 000 for polymyalgia rheumatica in people aged ≥50 years
- Possible cyclic pattern in incidence
- Siblings at increased risk

Clinical features[1]

1 Bilateral shoulder pain stiffness
2 Duration onset <2 weeks
3 Initial erythrocyte sedimentation rate >40 mm/hour
4 Stiffness >1 hour
5 Age >65 years
6 Depression or weight loss, or both
7 Bilateral upper arm tenderness

Probable PMR: 3 or more *or* <3 with clinical abnormality of temporal artery
Definite PMR: probable PMR responding to steroids

In polymyalgia rheumatica, the shoulder pain and stiffness are invariably bilateral, duration of onset relatively rapid, initial erythrocyte sedimentation rate usually high, and stiffness pronounced. Of the various systemic accompaniments, depression or weight loss, or both, are the most reliable. Sometimes, the muscles of the upper arms are tender on direct palpation, although muscle strength is usually unimpaired. Patients may have difficulty turning over in bed, particularly early in the morning. It may be hard to lift heavy objects, painful to walk up stairs, or tender to sit on the toilet. Patients comment on their "overwhelming illness." Upper arm tenderness when blood pressure is taken should raise suspicion.

Giant cell arteritis invariably presents with clinical features related to the affected arteries. In addition to fatigue, joint pain, and symptoms of polymyalgia rheumatica, headache and tenderness of the scalp are found, particularly around the temporal and occipital arteries. The scalp is tender to the touch, and it may hurt to wear spectacles. Clinical signs vary according to the duration of the disease. In the early stages, the pulse is full and bounding, and the arteries tender. Later, fibrosis and repair may predominate, and the pulse is almost absent. Diplopia, partial or complete loss of vision, and cranial nerve palsy may all occur if the condition remains untreated.

Polymyalgia: rarer mimics

- Polyarteritis nodosa
- Parkinson's disease
- Thyrotoxic myopathy
- Carcinomatous myopathy
- Systemic lupus erythematosus
- Pyrophosphate deposition
- Multiple myeloma
- Paget's disease
- Osteomalacia
- Polymyositis
- Malignancy

Polymyalgia: differential diagnosis

- Osteoarthritis
- Cervical spondylosis
- Frozen shoulder
- Rheumatoid arthritis

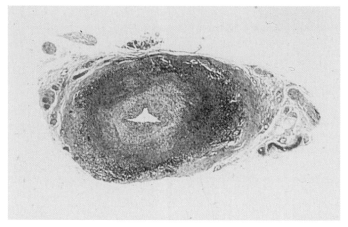

Histology of temporal arteritis (low power view). An inflammatory infiltrate is found in the media and intimal fibrosis. Luminal narrowing has occurred, so the artery is obliterated almost completely. Involvement of other arteries may occur, including the ophthalmic artery, which results in loss of vision

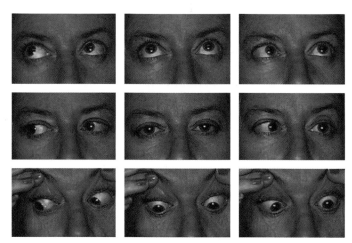

Temporary or permanent nerve palsy can occur in association with cranial arteritis. In this case the sixth nerve is clearly involved

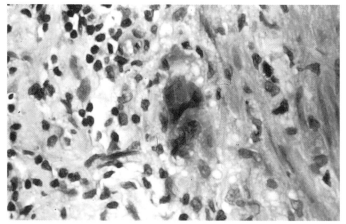

High powered view shows the inflammatory infiltrate complete with giant cells

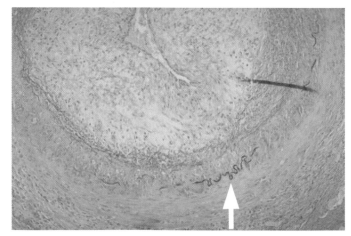

In this slide of giant cell arteritis elastic tissue appears black while various types of collagen stain yellow. Remnants of the internal elastic lamina are indicated by an arrow. Multi-nucleated giant cells and macrophages are attacking the elastic tissue and ingesting it. There is also extensive intimal proliferation and fibrosis

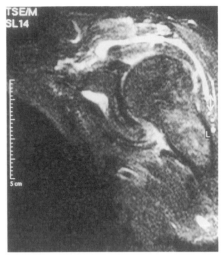
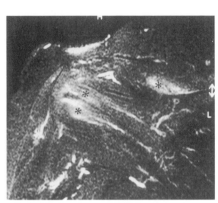
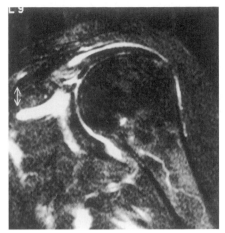

Magnetic resonance images of shoulder (T2 fat suppressed coronal oblique magnetic resonance imaging sequences) shows modest synovial inflammation with substantial fluid in the subacromial bursa associated with diffuse capsular oedema extending into the adjacent tendons and muscle bellies. Courtesy of Dr D McGonagle and Dr H Marzo-Ortega, Academic Unit of Musculoskeletal Disease, Leeds General Infirmary

Histopathology

Giant cell arteritis

The inflammatory features are typically described as illustrating the "skip" phenomenon due to the patchy or segmental involvement of the arteries. Giant cell arteritis is principally a disease driven by T cells that is limited to vessels with an internal elastic component. Histologically, the lesions are characterised by a mainly lymphocytic and macrophage infiltrate with the presence of giant and epithelioid cells. Essentially, the CD3+ T cell population comprises CD4+ or CD8+ subsets, of which CD4+ T cells predominate. The initial immunological event—the induction of CD4+ T cell proliferation by an unknown antigen—occurs in the outer vessel layer: the adventitia. These CD4 cells produce interferon γ, which attracts macrophages to the arterial wall where they fuse to form multinucleated giant cells in the intima–media junction. The giant cells produced express adhesion molecules, nitric oxide, and collagenases to result in, for example, tissue injury and in situ thrombosis.

Polymyalgia rheumatica

The histopathological features of polymyalgia rheumatica are defined less clearly. Several studies have confirmed their presence in about one third of patients with a non-erosive, self-limiting, asymmetrical arthritis (synovitis). The characteristics of synovitis on biopsy confirm a predominance of CD4+ T cells and macrophages. Similar to features described in giant cell arteritis, the vascular infiltrate reveals CD4+ interferon γ positive cells in the adventitia; macrophages that produce interleukin-1β, interleukin-6, endothelial cell adhesion molecules with matrix metalloproteinases, and inducible nitric oxide are seen in the media intima. Such temporal artery histology in patients with polymyalgia rheumatica has been seen in patients without the corresponding symptoms. Interestingly, magnetic resonance imaging studies also give evidence of an inflammatory process affecting distal articular or extra-articular (tenosynovial) structures, or both. Although skeletal muscle is not considered to be a site of pathology, focal changes in muscle ultrastructure and mitochondrial abnormalities have been noted, but the significance remains unclear. Muscle enzymes and biopsies are normal.

Investigations

Erythrocyte sedimentation rate is the most accepted and easily available marker, although polymyalgia rheumatica and even

---

Experimental markers of disease activity

- Interleukin-6
- Vascular endothelial growth factor
- Cytidine deaminase
- Activated CD8 lymphocytes
- Matrix metalloproteinase 9
- Monocyte chemoattractant protein-1
- YKL-40 (18-glycosyl hydrolase)
- Soluble interleukin-2 receptor

Accepted markers of disease activity

- Erythrocyte sedimentation rate
- C reactive protein
- Plasma viscosity

Biopsy for giant cell arteritis

- Biopsy is most useful just before or within 24 hours of treatment initiation with steroids, but treatment should not be delayed for the sake of obtaining a biopsy
- Skip lesions occur, so a negative result does not exclude giant cell arteritis
- A positive result may resolve later doubt about diagnosis, particularly if the response to treatment is not rapid and classical
- It is impossible to biopsy all patients, the decision depends on local resources
- One week after starting steroid treatment, the chance of obtaining positive biopsy falls to 10%

blindness from giant cell arteritis can occur in the presence of a normal erythrocyte sedimentation rate. The erythrocyte sedimentation rate, the C reactive protein, and the plasma viscosity all fall with effective treatment: the C reactive protein faster than the erythrocyte sedimentation rate or plasma viscosity. With treatment, normocytic normochromic anaemia corrects and a slight increase in hepatic alkaline phosphatase is reduced. In parallel, additional investigations should be arranged to exclude conditions that cause diagnostic confusion.

Treatment

Although some authors have suggested that a proportion of patients with polymyalgia rheumatica respond to non-steroidal anti-inflammatory drugs alone, treatment with corticosteroids is still mandatory, particularly when frequent visits can allow the dose to be accurately titrated against improvement and when additional prophylaxis for steroid complications, should they occur, is available. Data from the pre-steroid era suggest that untreated polymyalgia rheumatica and giant cell arteritis burn themselves out after a mean of two years (range six months to ten years).

Appropriate doses of steroids depend on the condition. Once a patient has been weaned off steroids at 2-3 years, it should be remembered that about 10% of patients will relapse within a ten-year period. Often the symptoms of relapse are more pronounced than the increase in acute phase reactants. In the case of relapse, the original dose of prednisolone should be reinstated.

For long-term therapy, the correct dose of steroids remains the lowest that keeps symptoms in complete remission, but if any doubt exists, a higher dose should be prescribed. Adverse events are best illustrated in the series from the Mayo clinic in which 232 patients received an average daily dose of 9.6 mg prednisolone for a mean duration of 2.4 years, 30 of the 232 having giant cell arteritis as well as polymyalgia rheumatica.[1] Cataracts occurred in 92 patients, hypertension in 43, and troublesome infection in 38. Diabetes was induced in 16 patients. Vertebral fracture occurred in 33 patients and fracture at another site in a further 32. Aseptic necrosis occurred in six patients and myopathy, which is hard to differentiate clinically from untreated polymyalgia rheumatica, in six. Prophylaxis for osteoporosis is necessary, particularly if treatment is of long duration and the patient not rendered mobile, or if other risk factors are present (see Chapter 10). It also remains important to check both cataract and hypertension.

Response criteria

The European Collaborating Polymyalgia Rheumatica Group recently proposed response criteria that aim to complement existing diagnostic criteria, as steroid response remains so important in diagnosis. It is also hoped that these will encourage the exploration of alternative drugs as steroid sparing agents when the need for steroids is persistent or when relapse occurs.

Steroid sparing agents

The evolution of steroid sparing agents for persistent disease has been somewhat disappointing. On current evidence, azathioprine probably remains the best choice. The reduction in prednisolone afforded by it is relatively small but clinically useful (mean of 1.9 mg/day rather than 4.2 mg/day at 52 weeks). The literature on the efficacy of methotrexate is conflicting;

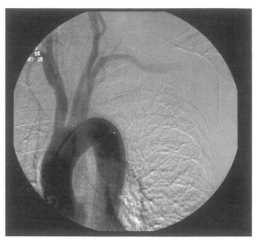

Arterial thrombosis complicating polymyalgia rheumatica, supporting a generalised vasculitic aetiology of this condition. Courtesy of Dr C Pease, Academic Unit of Musculoskeletal Disease, Leeds General Infirmary

---

Treatment of polymyalgia rheumatica

- Initial dose should be adjusted to patient's size and weight
- Typically start prednisolone 10-20 mg daily for one month
- After four weeks, aim to reduce the dose by 2.5 mg every 2-4 weeks, titrating against clinical response and level of acute phase reactants, with the aim of reducing to 10 mg/day
- After six months, try a further cautious reduction in increments of 1 mg/day every month in the hope of reducing to 5 mg/day, as long as symptoms do not recur
- Most patients require treatment for three years, but withdrawal over a period of some six months can be attempted at two years if the response has been good
- Some patients need up to ten years of treatment, and they may relapse

---

Treatment of giant cell arteritis

- Doses of prednisolone should be higher than for polymyalgia rheumatica and the period of treatment longer; the incentive to reduce is much less than with polymyalgia rheumatica
- For headaches alone, the starting dose of prednisolone should be in the range of 20-40 mg/day. With clinical signs of vasculitis or visual symptoms, the dose should be in the range of 40-60 mg/day. For impending or recent blindness, 80 mg/day should be given, possibly with the addition of intravenous hydrocortisone
- Dosage reduction can then be at the rate of about 5 mg every three or four weeks until a maintenance level of 10 or 15 mg/day is achieved, depending on response
- At one year, an effort should be made to reduce the dose to 5 mg/day in 1 mg steps
- Maintenance therapy at this low dose is likely to last up to five years

---

European Collaborating Polymyalgia Rheumatica Group's response criteria

Clinical improvement in pain (on visual analogue scale) and three out of four from:
- Reduction in C reactive protein or erythrocyte sedimentation rate, or both
- Improvement in morning stiffness
- Ability to raise shoulders
- Improvement on physicians' global assessment on visual analogue scale

most studies now suggest it does not provide a steroid sparing effect. The evidence for cyclosporin supports a steroid sparing effect, but some of the side effects summate with those of prednisolone. Efficacy for steroid sparing has also been claimed on behalf of dapsone, antimalarials, and cyclophosphamide. Theoretical reasons lead to a suspicion that modification of interleukins might be helpful. This might be achieved by using drugs to block tumour necrosis factor α or drugs yet to be marketed to block interleukin-6. The use of such drugs remains experimental at present.

1 Gabriel SE, Sunku J, Salvarani C, O'fallon WM, Hunder GG. Adverse outcomes of antiinflammatory therapy among patients with polymyalgia rheumatica. *Arthritis Rheum* 1997;40:1873-8

Reviews

- Salvarani C, Cantini F, Boiardi L, Hunder GG. Polymyalgia rheumatica and giant-cell arteritis. *N Eng J Med* 2002;347:261-71
- Levine SM, Hellmann DB. Giant-cell arteritis. *Curr Opin Rheumatol* 2002;14:3-10
- Hunder GG. Clinical features of GCA/PMR. *Clin Exp Rheumatol* 2000;18:56-8
- Swannell AJ. Polymyalgia rheumatica and temporal arteritis: diagnosis and management. *BMJ* 1997;31:1329-32
- Genetic and environmental factors in polymyalgia rheumatica. *Ann Rheum Dis* 1997;56:576-7

Text on clinical improvement in pain courtesy of Dr Burkhard Leeb. The photographs of the histology of temporal arthritis, sixth nerve palsy, inflammatory infiltrate with giant cells are reproduced with permission from Bhatti T. *The neuro-ophthalmic manifestations of giant cell arthritis—an interactive tutorial* (www.medinfo.ufl.edu/cme/grounds/bhatti/index.html). They are copyright of the University of Florida. The photograph of giant cells and macrophages attacking elastic tissue is reproduced from Schmidt R, et al. *Systemic pathology—an interactive tutorial* (www.eduserv.hscer.washington.edu/hubio546/jpgs575/spd/ img0021.jpg). It is copyright of the University of Washington.

Use of steroid sparing agents

If steroid treatment is prolonged or if substantial side effects occur, consider the addition of one of the following:
- Azathioprine
- Methotrexate
- Cyclosporin
- Tumour necrosis factor α blockade

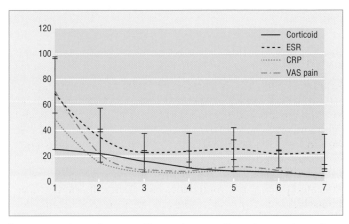

Improvement in erythrocyte sedimentation rate, C reactive protein, and the patient's perception of pain (measured on a visual analogue scale) in response to corticosteroid therapy in a group of 76 patients with polymyalgia rheumatica. Courtesy of Dr Burkhard Leeb

16 Systemic lupus erythematosus, antiphospholipid antibody syndrome, and other lupus-like syndromes

Tsui-Yee Lian, Caroline Gordon

Systemic lupus erythematosus is a multisystemic autoimmune disease of unknown cause with a wide variety of manifestations, which is often characterised by remissions and relapses. Systemic lupus erythematosus is part of a spectrum of autoimmune diseases that includes neonatal lupus, Sjögren's syndrome, antiphospholipid antibody, and overlap syndromes. Antiphospholipid antibody may occur as a primary disorder or secondary to systemic lupus erythematosus or another autoimmune condition, such as autoimmune hypothyroidism or chronic active hepatitis.[1] As no cure exists for these conditions, life-long follow up is needed, so it is important that the primary care physician, patient, and hospital specialists are involved closely in the management of these diseases.

Cause

Systemic lupus erythematosus is a multifactorial disease. The disease is characterised by the development of autoantibodies, and increasing evidence shows that autoantibodies may arise from failed clearance of apoptotic cells. The potential mechanisms have been reviewed recently.[8] Much of the disease is due to deposition of immune complexes and the activation of complement. Antiphospholipid antibodies are a specific family of autoantibodies directed against anionic phospholipids that are located in cell membranes. The pathogenic mechanisms in antiphospholipid syndrome relate to the prothrombotic effects of these antibodies in vivo.

Epidemiology

The prevalence of systemic lupus erythematosus depends on the country and ethnic mix of the population. It is more common in women and black people. Some studies have suggested that systemic lupus erythematosus is more common in the East and in Chinese people. In Malaysia, where there was an ethnic mix of 53% Malays, 36% Chinese, and 11% Indians in the 1970s, most admissions for systemic lupus erythematosus were of Chinese people (81%).[4] This may reflect more severe disease in Chinese people.

Clinical presentations

Systemic lupus erythematosus
The American Rheumatology Association's 1982 classification criteria for systemic lupus erythematosus were revised in 1997. These criteria were designed not for diagnosis but for classifying patients into studies and clinical trials. The diagnosis of systemic lupus erythematosus should be considered if a patient has characteristic features of lupus, even if they do not fulfil four of the eleven criteria. For example, a 25 year old woman with malar rash, positive antinuclear antibody, and histologically proven glomerulonephritis obviously has systemic lupus erythematosus, despite fulfilling only three criteria.

Prevalence of systemic lupus erythematosus[2–6]

Population and country of origin	Prevalence (per 100 000)
United Kingdom	
• Adults	27.7
• Women	49.6
	(one per 2000 women)
• Caucasians	20.7
• Afro-Caribbeans	111.8
• Asians (from Indian subcontinent)	46.7
Singaporean adults	33
Vietnamese	42
Taiwanese adults	33

Factors involved in systemic lupus erythematosus

- Genetic factors[7]
  - Major histocompatibility complex class II antigen DR3
  - Genes for complement
  - Receptors for Fc gamma II and III
- Environmental triggers
  - Ultraviolet light
  - Drug exposure
- Infections
  - Viruses
- Hormonal factors
  - Oestrogens

American Rheumatology Association's revised classification criteria for systemic lupus erythematosus

Patients should have experienced at least four of the following criteria at some point in their disease course to be classified as suffering from systemic lupus erythematosus:

- Malar rash
- Discoid rash
- Photosensitivity
- Oral ulcers
- Arthritis
- Serositis
- Renal disorder
- Neurological disorder
- Haematological disorder
- Immunological disorder
- Positive antinuclear antibodies

Cumulative percentage incidence of clinical features of systemic lupus erythematosus[9]

Feature	Indian (%)	Western (%)
Arthritis	72-92	86-94
Alopecia	52-80	50
Skin rash	74-90	60
Photosensitivity	10-62	33-62
Malar rash	37-76	72-90
Oral ulcers	41-61	30
Fever	74-91	80
Neuropsychiatric	19-63	20-45
Renal	35-73	29-73
Cardiac	10-29	20-30
Pleuropulmonary	9-54	36-57

Systemic lupus erythematosus, antiphospholipid antibody syndrome, and other lupus-like syndromes

General features

Fatigue is common, troublesome, and difficult to evaluate. It may be associated with depression or fibromyalgia secondary to systemic lupus erythematosus, hypothyroidism (often autoimmune in nature), anaemia, or cardiovascular problems. Other constitutional symptoms of active disease include fever, malaise, anorexia, and weight loss.

Mucocutaneous manifestations

The most common mucocutaneous features are painful or painless mouth ulcers, diffuse alopecia, butterfly or malar rash, and photosensitivity. Nasal or vaginal ulcers may also occur. Mucocutaneous features are more prominent in Asians and whites. Subacute cutaneous lupus erythematosus is a non-scarring rash that is found in areas of the body exposed to the sun. Discoid lesions are chronic scarring lesions. Non-scarring alopecia may be patchy or diffuse. Rapid, spontaneous hair loss indicates active disease. Raynaud's phenomenon is usually milder than in scleroderma.

Musculoskeletal manifestations

Generalised arthralgia with early morning stiffness and no swelling is very common. A non-erosive arthritis with joint tenderness and swelling may develop. Deformities are unusual but may occur due to ligamentous laxity (Jacoud's arthropathy). Myalgia is common but inflammatory myositis occurs in only 5% of patients. Myopathy can be caused by corticosteroids, antimalarials, and lipid lowering agents. Avascular necrosis and infection should be suspected if the patient complains of sudden onset, severe pain in only one joint.

Haematological manifestations

Leucopenia may be an early clue to the diagnosis of systemic lupus erythematosus. Lymphopenia is the most common manifestation of systemic lupus erythematosus other than positive antinuclear antibodies and, in untreated patients, is caused by lymphocytotoxic antibodies. Mild neutropenia is relatively common in black people even without systemic lupus erythematosus, but values $< 1.5 \times 10^9/l$ are usually related to disease or drugs. Thrombocytopenia may occur as an immune mediated condition associated with a risk of bleeding, as in idiopathic thrombocytopenic purpura, or as a milder abnormality with platelet counts $> 80 \times 10^9/l$ associated with a risk of thrombosis in the antiphospholipid syndrome (see below).

Renal manifestations

Renal disease is an important determinant of the outcome of systemic lupus erythematosus.[10] Early nephritis is often asymptomatic, so regular urinalysis for protein, blood, and casts is essential. Some patients present with nephrotic syndrome and a few with devastating accelerated hypertension and renal shutdown. Renal biopsy is helpful for assessing the severity, nature, extent, and reversibility of the involvement and is an important guide to treatment and prognosis.

Nervous system manifestations

Systemic lupus erythematosus may affect the central and peripheral nervous systems. Definitions for these manifestations have been proposed by a consensus group.[11] The most common manifestations are headache, seizures, aseptic meningitis, and cerebrovascular accidents. Antiphospholipid antibodies (including anticardiolipin antibodies) have been implicated in cerebrovascular accidents and chorea. It often is hard to determine whether the depression and headaches are due to lupus itself; in many cases, they are related to psychosocial issues. Other possible causes such as sepsis, drugs, uraemia,

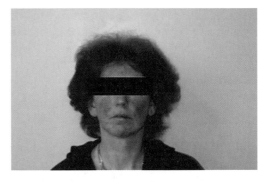

Malar rash in systemic lupus erythematosus

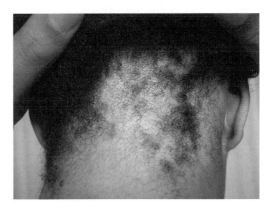

Patient with patchy alopecia

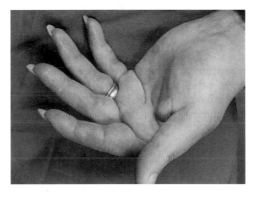

Jacoud's arthropathy

The most common form of anaemia is a normochromic normocytic anaemia of chronic disease. Some patients develop an antibody mediated haemolytic anaemia and others an iron deficiency anaemia secondary to peptic ulceration or gastritis (usually due to non-steroidal anti-inflammatory drugs)

Central nervous system manifestations of systemic lupus erythematosus

- Aseptic meningitis
- Cerebrovascular disease
- Demyelinating syndrome
- Headache (including migraine and benign intracranial hypertension)
- Movement disorders (including chorea)
- Myelopathy
- Seizure disorders
- Acute confusional state
- Anxiety disorder
- Cognitive dysfunction
- Mood disorder
- Psychosis

severe hypertension, and other metabolic causes must be sought and treated. Steroids are often blamed for inducing psychosis, but if any doubt exists, patients should be given more, not less, steroid while under medical supervision, particularly if active lupus is evident in other systems.

Pulmonary and cardiovascular manifestations

Pleurisy, often without physical signs, is common in systemic lupus erythematosus. Less common manifestations are lupus pneumonitis, pulmonary haemorrhage, pulmonary embolism, and pulmonary hypertension. Pulmonary haemorrhage can be sudden and acute and has high mortality. Pulmonary hypertension is associated with a poor prognosis, especially in pregnancy. Pericarditis is common but often asymptomatic. Other cardiac manifestations are myocarditis and endocarditis. Coronary artery disease is occasionally caused by vasculitis, but more often results from premature atherosclerosis.

Gastrointestinal manifestations

Abdominal pain, nausea, vomiting, and diarrhoea occur in up to 50% of patients at some stage of disease.[12] Although the presentation of greatest importance is mesenteric vasculitis, in which the patient presents with an acute abdomen and is at high risk of death, there have been recent reports of patients with subacute abdominal pain or aseptic peritonitis. This is usually associated with other serological signs of active disease and generally improves with steroid therapy.[14] Other abdominal manifestations include subacute bowel obstruction,[15] hepatitis, sclerosing cholangitis, protein losing enteropathy, pancreatitis, and ascites. Exclusion or treatment of infection is essential in patients with these conditions.

Pregnancy and systemic lupus erythematosus

No evidence suggests that systemic lupus erythematosus reduces fertility, but active disease and the presence of antiphospholipid antibody syndrome (see below) may increase the risk of intrauterine growth retardation, premature delivery, miscarriages, and stillbirth. Doses of prednisolone >10 mg/day predispose to pre-eclampsia, isolated hypertension in pregnancy, premature rupture of membranes, and maternal infection. No evidence shows that prednisolone crosses the placenta and causes fetal abnormalities in humans. Increasing evidence shows that azathioprine (<2 mg/kg/day) and hydroxychloroquine (200 mg daily) can be continued in pregnancy. Pulmonary hypertension is associated with a 50% risk of mortality, particularly in the first 72 hours after delivery.[16] This is usually a contraindication to planned pregnancy and needs specialist multidisciplinary care if diagnosed in pregnancy.

Neonatal lupus syndrome

This is a syndrome that occurs in about 10% of babies born to mothers with anti-Ro or anti-La antibodies. The most common manifestation is a rash induced by ultraviolet light a few days after birth. It resolves spontaneously if the babies are removed from sunlight or ultraviolet light. A more serious, but much rarer, manifestation of this syndrome is congenital heart block. This is usually detected in utero about 16-28 weeks into the pregnancy.

Sjögren's syndrome

This clinical syndrome is characterised by sicca symptoms: dry eyes and dry mouth due to failure of salivary and mucosal glands, often preceded by salivary gland swelling. It may occur

---

Peripheral nervous system manifestations of systemic lupus erythematosus

- Acute inflammatory demyelinating polyradiculoneuropathy (Guillain-Barré syndrome)
- Autonomic disorder
- Mononeuropathy (single or multiplex)
- Myasthenia gravis
- Neuropathy, cranial
- Plexopathy
- Polyneuropathy

Survival and disease control have improved in patients with systemic lupus erythematosus, but complications of premature vascular disease are recognised increasingly: the relative risk for myocardial infarction in women with systemic lupus erythematosus aged 35-44 years was 52.3 times the risk for women without lupus[13]

Pregnant women with lupus need close monitoring for optimal fetal and maternal outcome and are best managed in specialist units

---

Most babies born with congenital heart block need a pacemaker during the first year of life

as a secondary disorder in patients with systemic lupus erythematosus or other conditions, including rheumatoid arthritis, systemic sclerosis, and primary biliary cirrhosis, or as a primary disorder with features that resemble a mild form of systemic lupus erythematosus (mild symmetrical arthritis, photosensitivity, fatigue, and diffuse alopecia). The primary syndrome is associated with hypergammaglobulinaemia with very high total immunoglobulin G levels and positive antinuclear antibody, rheumatoid factor, and anti-Ro and anti-La antibody tests. Hydroxychloroquine and pilocarpine with other local symptomatic measures, such as artificial tears, are used to treat the condition.

> **Sjögren's syndrome is often misdiagnosed as rheumatoid arthritis or systemic lupus erythematosus**

Overlap syndromes and other lupus-like conditions

Up to 25% of patients with connective tissue disorders do not fit into classical descriptions and present with overlapping clinical features.[17] Some may evolve into well defined connective tissue disorders, while others have manifestations of more than one definite connective tissue disorders—for example, systemic sclerosis combined with systemic lupus erythematosus and inflammatory myositis (see Chapter 18). Raynaud's phenomenon is often present and may occur in isolation as the first manifestation of a connective tissue disorder. Patients with mild undifferentiated connective tissue disorders may have inflammatory arthritis, oedema of hands, and acrosclerosis. Generally prognosis is good as long as patients do not develop pulmonary hypertension.

Antiphospholipid syndrome

Antiphospholipid syndrome is an important cause of recurrent arterial and venous thrombosis and miscarriages.[11]

Thrombosis

The most common presentation of antiphospholipid syndrome is venous thrombosis in the arms or legs, which is often recurrent, multiple, and bilateral, with a propensity for pulmonary embolism. Arterial thrombosis is less common but most frequently manifested by features of ischaemia or infarction. The severity of presentation depends on the acuteness and extent of the occlusion. The brain is the most common site, where thrombosis presents as stroke and transient ischaemic attacks. Other sites for arterial occlusion are the coronary arteries, subclavian, renal, retinal, and pedal arteries.

Obstetric syndromes

Recurrent pregnancy losses in the second or third trimester are typical. Patients should be monitored for intrauterine growth retardation due to placental insufficiency and pre-eclampsia in a specialist unit. Planned early delivery is often required.

Other manifestations

Other prominent features include thrombocytopenia (up to 50% of patients), haemolytic anaemia, livedo reticularis, chronic ulcers, typically near the medial malleolus, and cutaneous vasculitis.

Catastrophic antiphospholipid syndrome

This is an acute and devastating syndrome characterised by multiple simultaneous vascular occlusions throughout the body, that are often fatal. The kidney is affected most

---

Criteria for classification of antiphospholipid syndrome

Clinical features

Thrombosis
- Confirmed episode of arterial and/or venous thrombosis in any organ or tissue

Morbidity in pregnancy
- Fetal death beyond ten weeks' gestation with confirmed normal fetal morphology
- Three or more spontaneous abortions before ten weeks' gestation in the absence of other maternal causes
- More than one premature birth due to presence of severe placental insufficiency, pre-eclampsia or eclampsia before 34 weeks' gestation

Laboratory criteria
- Immunoglobulin G and/or immunoglobulin M anticardiolipin antibodies in medium to high titre on at least two different occasions more than six weeks apart (using a standard enzyme-linked immunosorbent assay for β_2-glycoprotein I dependent anticardiolipin antibodies)
- Lupus anticoagulant in plasma on two separate occasions at least six weeks apart

Antiphospholipid syndrome definitely is present if at least one of the clinical features and one of the laboratory criteria are met.

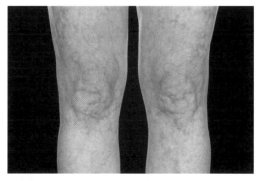

Livedo reticularis

often, followed by the lungs, central nervous system, heart, and skin.

Outcome of systemic lupus erythematosus and antiphospholipid syndrome

Although survival has improved substantially over the last 50 years (90% of patients survive at least five years and over 80% at least ten years), awareness is increasing that these patients succumb to late complications of the disease or its therapy.[13] In particular, hyperlipidaemia, hypertension, premature ischaemic heart disease, diabetes mellitus, and osteoporotic fractures may develop. Compliance with medications, clinic visits, and lifestyle modifications is essential to prevent or reduce the risk of these associated problems, which may be iatrogenic or disease related in origin. The long-term prognosis of antiphospholipid syndrome is poor, with organ damage in about one third and functional impairment in up to one fifth of patients at the end of ten years.[18]

Investigations

Investigations in systemic lupus erythematosus
A full blood count with differential white count, urinalysis and serum creatinine should be done for diagnosis and monitoring of the activity of systemic lupus erythematosus. Creatinine clearance or other assessment of glomerular filtration rate is more reliable for detecting early impairment of renal function. Patients with proteinuria or haematuria, or both, on dipstick must have microscopy done to look for casts if infection, stones, and menstrual blood loss have been excluded.

For diagnosis, antinuclear antibody and anti-extractable nuclear antigens tests (see Chapter 20) should be done. No value is gained by repeating these tests, unless a change in clinical features is noted. Anti-ribonucleoprotein is associated with mixed connective tissue disease. Anti-dsDNA antibodies are useful for predicting patients at risk of developing renal disease and for monitoring disease activity. Although levels usually rise before a disease flare, they may fall at the time of flare. Levels of C3 and C4 fall with disease activity because of complement consumption, particularly in patients with renal disease. Levels also relate to the rate of synthesis in the liver and may rise in infections and pregnancy. Measurement of complement degradation products (for example, C3d, C4d) is less widely available but is more reliable for monitoring disease activity, as these reflect complement consumption alone. In women who are planning pregnancy, it is important to check for anti-Ro and anti-La antibodies and for antiphospholipid antibodies.

Investigations in antiphospholipid syndrome[19]
Overall, 80-90% of patients with antiphospholipid syndrome are positive for antibodies to a complex of anticardiolipin antibodies and β_2-glycoprotein I. Lupus anticoagulant is only found in 20% of patients with antiphospholipid syndrome but is associated with a high risk of thrombosis. Low levels of antiphospholipid antibodies of no clinical consequence may develop transiently after infections.

Tests for antiphospholipid antibodies
- Anticardiolipin antibodies
- Antibodies against cofactors associated with anionic phospholipids, for example, β_2-glycoprotein I
- Lupus anticoagulant
- Biological false positive serological tests for syphilis

Management of systemic lupus erythematosus
- Avoid sun and other ultraviolet light
- Wear sun block
- Avoid infection
- Treat bacterial infections early with antibiotics
- Avoid unplanned pregnancy
- Advise appropriate contraception
- Use non-steroidal anti-inflammatory drugs with care
- Use other analgesics as needed
- Use oral steroids with care
- Consider local and intramuscular or intravenous steroids and cytotoxic agents
- Monitor for active disease
- Urinalysis, full blood count, creatinine, anti-dsDNA antibodies, C3, C4
- Screen for hypertension
- Treat with calcium channel blockers or angiotensin-converting enzyme inhibitors
- Screen for diabetes and lipids
- Advise on diet and give drugs if needed
- Assess osteoporosis risk
- Give postmenopausal women bisphosphonates

Tests for antiphospholipid antibodies must be positive on two separate occasions, at least six weeks apart, before a confident diagnosis of antiphospholipid syndrome can be made

Management

General measures

Patients must be educated about the nature of their disease and the need for therapy. Leaflets from patient support organisations and references to reliable internet websites are useful. More than just drug therapy is required. Patients with sun-induced rashes should use sunblock regularly for about six months over the summer. Other patients with systemic lupus erythematosus should be aware that sun exposure may precipitate a disease flare.

Infections should be avoided and treated promptly if appropriate, as they can precipitate flares. Similarly, contraceptive pills that contain oestrogen may exacerbate lupus disease or thrombosis and should be used with caution. In general, barrier methods or progesterone-only contraception are preferred. Pregnancy should be planned, as the outcome is better, with fewer complications in both mother and fetus, if the mother has inactive disease at the time of conception. Drug therapy should be reviewed before conception.

Overlap and lupus-like conditions are managed much the same as mild systemic lupus erythematosus. Dry eyes should be managed by the frequent use of artificial tears. Dry mouth is best managed by taking sips of plain water, sucking ice cubes, or eating sugar free sweets. Artificial saliva preparations are disappointing.

Drug therapy in systemic lupus erythematosus

Milder cases with intermittent rashes, arthritis, and other mucocutaneous features can usually be treated with steroid creams, non-steroidal anti-inflammatory drugs, and hydroxychloroquine (<6.5 mg/kg/day). These drugs are also widely used in overlap syndromes, with the exception of non-steroidal anti-inflammatory drugs, which are contraindicated in patients with systemic sclerosis. More persistent cases of systemic lupus erythematosus may need oral corticosteroids. Patients who need 10 mg/day of prednisolone or more despite hydroxychloroquine, or those who present with more severe manifestations that need higher initial doses of prednisolone (0.5-1 mg/kg/day), may need azathioprine, methotrexate, or cyclosporin A as steroid sparing immunosuppressive agents. Non-steroidal anti-inflammatory drugs should not be used in patients with renal disease. Steroids should always be reduced slowly.

Mycophenolate mofetil is a promising alternative drug for the treatment of severe lupus. In pregnancy and breastfeeding, patients may be given prednisolone. Azathioprine and hydroxychloroquine rarely cause problems at low doses, but some doctors prefer to avoid them altogether. Methotrexate and cyclophosphamide are contraindicated in pregnancy and while breastfeeding. Cyclosporin A has been used in pregnancy in patients who have undergone transplants, but it is not yet recommended in pregnancies in those with systemic lupus erythematosus.

Meticulous screening for blood pressure control, treatment of diabetes and hyperlipidaemia, and prophylaxis for steroid induced osteoporosis are essential. In general, calcium channel blockers and angiotensin converting enzyme inhibitors are the preferred antihypertensive agents, because β blockers aggravate Raynaud's phenomenon.

Bisphosphonates are often required in postmenopausal women, but they should be used with great care in women who may want to become pregnant in the future. Hormone

> **Lifestyle should be adjusted to ensure adequate rest, appropriate exercise, and a well balanced diet. Measures for reducing stress should be considered and career plans reviewed. Patients with Raynaud's phenomenon should wear appropriate warm clothing, including hats and gloves**

Steroid sparing and cytotoxic drugs used in systemic lupus erythematosus

Drug	Dose range (mg/kg/day)
Hydroxychloroquine	≤ 6.5
Azathioprine	1-2.5
Methotrexate	7.5-25 mg per week
Cyclosporin A	1-2.5
Cyclophosphamide	Intravenous pulses or ≤ 2 mg/kg/day orally
Mycophenolate mofetil	1-3 g/day

> **Cyclophosphamide is often given as intermittent intravenous "pulse therapy" and is used predominantly for proliferative glomerulonephritis and systemic vasculitis**

> **Raynaud's phenomenon is best treated with calcium channel blockers, local nitrate creams if mild to moderate, and intravenous prostacyclin infusions in severe cases. Angiotensin converting enzyme inhibitors may be tried if calcium channel blockers are not tolerated**

replacement therapy should be used with care and is contraindicated in women with antiphospholipid antibodies who are not anticoagulated. Calcium and vitamin D can be used in all age groups. Treatment with anticoagulation and antiepileptic, antidepressant, or antipsychotic drugs should be considered early in the management of patients with neuropsychiatric disease. Analgesics and antimigraine drugs are used for headache.

Therapy in antiphospholipid antibody syndrome
There is no recommendation for prophylactic treatment of patients serologically positive for antiphospholipid antibody syndrome but without a history of thrombosis. Treatment for thrombosis is usually initiated with intravenous or subcutaneous heparin and is soon changed to oral anticoagulation with warfarin—as for any other acute thrombosis. Most doctors recommend maintaining the international normalised ratio at about 3.5 to prevent further thrombosis.[11] Anticoagulation should be life-long unless a contraindication is present. Corticosteroids and immunosuppressive drugs are not recommended in patients with antiphospholipid antibody syndrome unless needed for other manifestations of lupus.

Goals of treatment in antiphospholipid syndrome
- Prophylaxis
- Treatment of acute thromboses
- Prevention of further thrombotic events
- Management of pregnancy in antiphospholipid syndrome

Pregnancy
A combination of low molecular weight heparin and low dose aspirin is preferred.[20] Pregnant women need close monitoring by the obstetrician, haematologist, and rheumatologist, preferably in combined clinics at specialist units.

Conclusion

Systemic lupus erythematosus is more common than many people realise. The presentations are diverse, and it may take a few years to realise that a variety of symptoms and signs can all be attributed to systemic lupus erythematosus, Sjögren's syndrome, or an overlap syndrome. Antiphospholipid antibody syndrome should be sought actively in patients with a history of recurrent miscarriages or thrombosis, or both, because of the risk of future thrombotic complications. With appropriate treatment, the outcome of these conditions is good, but the risk of late complications, particularly those of a vascular nature, is important. In future, the management of patients with these conditions should seek to reduce these risks as well as control active disease.

1 Asherson RA, Cervera R. "Primary", "secondary" and other variants of the antiphospholipid syndrome. *Lupus* 1994;3:293-8
2 Johnson AE, Gordon C, Palmer RG, Bacon PA. The prevalence and incidence of systemic lupus erythematosus in Birmingham, England. Relationship to ethnicity and country of birth. *Arthritis Rheum* 1995;38:551-8
3 Boey M. Systemic lupus erythematosus. In: Wei-Howe K, Pao-Hsii F, eds. *Textbook of clinical rheumatology*. Singapore: National Arthritis Foundation of Singapore; 1997:17-29
4 Frank AO. Apparent predisposition to systemic lupus erythematosus in Chinese patients in West Malaysia. *Ann Rheum Dis* 1980;39:266-9
5 Phan JC, Bush TM, Donald F, Ward M. Clinical and laboratory features of patients of Vietnamese descent with systemic lupus erythematosus. *Lupus* 1999;8:521-4
6 Chou CT, Pei L, Chang DM, Lee CF, Schumacher HR, Liang MH. Prevalence of rheumatic diseases in Taiwan: a population study of urban, surburban, rural differences. *J Rheumatol* 1994;21:302-6
7 Tan FK, Arnett FC. The genetics of lupus. *Curr Opin Rheumatol* 1998;10:399-408
8 Gordon C, Salmon M. Update on systemic lupus erythematosus: autoantibodies and apoptosis. *Clin Med* 2001;1:10-14
9 Joshi VR. Systemic lupus erythematosus. In: Pispati P, ed. *Manual of Rheumatology*. Mumbai: Indian Rheumatology Association, 2002:177-89
10 Stoll T, Seifert B, Isenberg DA. SLICC/ACR damage index is valid, and renal and pulmonary organ scores are predictors of severe outcome in patients with systemic lupus erythematosus. *Br J Rheumatol* 1996;35:248-54
11 Ruiz-Irastorza G, Khamashta MA, Castellino G, Hughes GRV. Systemic lupus erythematosus. *Lancet* 2001;357:1027-32
12 Medina F, Ayala A, Jara LJ, Becerra M, Miranda JM, Fraga A. Acute abdomen in systemic lupus erythematosus: the importance of early laparotomy. *Am J Med* 1997;103:100-5
13 Gordon C. Long-term complications of systemic lupus erythematosus. *Rheumatology* 2002;41:1095-100
14 Buck AC, Serebro LH, Quinet RJ. Subacute abdominal pain requiring hospitalization in a systemic lupus erythematosus patient: a retrospective analysis and review of the literature. *Lupus* 2001;10:491-5
15 Mok MY, Wong RW, Lau CS. Intestinal pseudo-obstruction in systemic lupus erythematosus: an uncommon but important clinical manifestation. *Lupus* 2000;9:11-18
16 Martin WL, Gordon C, Kilby MD. Systemic lupus erythematosus. *Lancet* 2001;358:586
17 Maddison P. Overlap syndromes. In: Wei-Howe K, Pao-Hsii F, eds. *Textbook of clinical rheumatology*. Singapore: National Arthritis Foundation of Singapore; 1997:332-53
18 Erkan D, Yazici Y, Sobel R, Lockshin MD. Primary antiphospholipid syndrome: functional outcome after 10 years. *J Rheumatol* 2000;27:2817-21
19 Petri M. Diagnosis of antiphospholipid antibodies. *Rheum Dis Clin North Am* 1994;20:443-69
20 Kutteh WH. Antiphospholipid antibody-associated recurrent pregnancy loss: treatment with heparin and low-dose aspirin is superior to low-dose aspirin alone. *Am J Obstet Gynecol* 1996;174:1584-9

17 Raynaud's phenomenon and scleroderma

Christopher P Denton, Carol M Black

Spectrum of scleroderma

Scleroderma, meaning "hard skin", is a generic term used to describe related connective tissue disorders. The spectrum ranges from localised dermal sclerosis, through systemic conditions that feature cutaneous and internal organ fibrosis together with vascular dysfunction, to the purely vascular disorders of Raynaud's phenomenon. These conditions overlap clinically and pathologically. Important differential diagnoses exist for each group of conditions, although, like scleroderma itself, they are rare.

Raynaud's phenomenon

Implications

Episodic cold-induced vasospasm triggered by cold or emotional stress affects around 5% of the adult population, especially young women. Primary Raynaud's (90%) needs no other clinical or investigational abnormalities, but secondary Raynaud's (10%) is suggestive of other features, usually an underlying autoimmune rheumatic disease. Investigation of Raynaud's symptoms includes identification of secondary causes. Such causes of Raynaud's or acrocyanosis include vibrating machine tools, thoracic outlet obstruction, drugs such as β blockers, and haematological abnormalities such as cryoglobulinaemia. Macrovascular arterial disease, embolisation, and systemic vasculitis, such as Berger's disease, are important but rare differential diagnoses. Some patients with Raynaud's phenomenon have no other clinical abnormalities but have positive autoantibodies, especially antinuclear antibodies, with evidence of microvasculopathy in nailfold capillaries. This group of patients includes those who will develop significant connective tissue disease within the next 5-10 years. The frequency of this transition is about 10%. The negative predictive value of normal nailfold capillaroscopy and negative autoantibody screening is powerful and allows robust reassurance. Benign primary Raynaud's must be distinguished from more serious conditions with possible implications for life insurance and mortgage protection policies, for example.

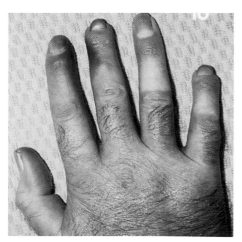

Well defined blanching of skin characteristic of Raynaud's phenomenon

---

Spectrum of scleroderma and scleroderma-like disorders

Scleroderma

Localised scleroderma
- Dermal inflammation and fibrosis
- No visceral disease and few vascular symptoms

Plaque morphoea
- Fewer than four localised areas of involvement

Generalised morphoea
- More than four areas or widespread lesions

Linear scleroderma
- Skin sclerosis follows dermatomal distribution
- Most common form of childhood onset scleroderma

En coup de sabre
- Scalp and facial linear lesion often with underlying bone changes

Systemic sclerosis

Diffuse cutaneous systemic sclerosis
- Skin involvement proximal to elbows or knees
- Short history of Raynaud's phenomenon
- Associated with anti-scl70 or anti-RNA polymerase antibodies

Limited cutaneous systemic sclerosis
- Skin tightening affects extremities only
- Long history of Raynaud's phenomenon
- Associated with anti-centromere autoantibodies

Overlap syndromes
- Clinical features of scleroderma associated with those of another autoimmune rheumatic disease (systemic lupus erythematosus, myositis, and arthritis)

Systemic sclerosis sine scleroderma
- Serological, vascular, and visceral features of scleroderma without detectable skin sclerosis

Isolated Raynaud's phenomenon

Primary
- Common, onset in adolescence, female predominance, normal nailfold capillaroscopy, and negative autoantibody profile

Secondary
- Raynaud's phenomenon with abnormal nailfold capillaries or positive autoantibody testing, or both

---

Points to consider when looking for underlying cause of Raynaud's phenomenon

- Occupation
    - Working outdoors
    - Fishing industry
    - Using vibrating tools
    - Exposure to chemicals such as vinyl chloride
- Examination of peripheral and central vascular system for proximal vascular occlusion
- Drugs
    - β blockers
    - Oral contraceptives
    - Bleomycin
    - Migraine therapy
- Symptoms of other autoimmune rheumatic disorders
    - Arthralgia or arthritis
    - Cerebral symptoms
    - Mouth ulcers
    - Alopecia
    - Photosensitivity
    - Muscle weakness
    - Skin rashes
    - Dry eyes or mouth
    - Respiratory or cardiac problems

Associations

Many patients with a defined connective tissue disease have Raynaud's phenomenon. For systemic sclerosis, 95% of patients have Raynaud's phenomenon, and this emphasises a likely central role for vascular abnormalities. In lupus, polymyositis, or dermatomyositis, the frequency of Raynaud's is around 50%. It is less common in other diseases, including Sjogren's syndrome and rheumatoid arthritis. Many patients with overlap syndromes have Raynaud's phenomenon and also features such as arthralgia, malaise, or photosensitivity, but do not fulfil classification criteria for a defined disease. These are best described as cases of undifferentiated connective tissue disease, which may later evolve into more significant diseases (see also Chapters 18 and 20).

Controversy surrounds patients with hallmark autoantibodies of scleroderma in association with Raynaud's. Potentially some of these may have, or develop, scleroderma sine scleroderma with major visceral fibrosis; another subgroup seems to have minor features of scleroderma. The term "limited scleroderma" has been proposed recently, but has not been adopted universally. Until the natural history of these individuals is better defined, it is important that they be clearly distinguished from scleroderma for management.

Systemic sclerosis

The most severe forms of scleroderma are within the systemic sclerosis subgroup. Most cases fall into two major subsets. The diffuse cutaneous subset is determined by involvement of skin proximal to the knees and elbows and may be confused with inflammatory arthropathy in its early stages. Most of the important complications develop within the first three years of diffuse cutaneous scleroderma, and skin sclerosis tends to be maximal at around 18-30 months. After this time, involvement of the skin tends to stabilise or improve. Diffuse cutaneous scleroderma is not usually a two phase illness, although important organ based complications and co-morbidity can be clinically more significant later. Raynaud's phenomenon generally develops concurrently with skin disease or shortly afterwards. The limited cutaneous subset of scleroderma accounts for around 60% of cases in most North American or European series. Skin involvement is much less extensive and may be confined to the fingers (sclerodactyly), face, or neck. Raynaud's phenomenon is very prominent and may precede development of scleroderma by several years.

The designation of "CREST" syndrome is popular in the United States and refers to a subgroup of limited cutaneous scleroderma, in which **c**alcinosis, **R**aynaud's phenomenon, o**e**sophageal dysmotility, **s**clerodactyly, and **t**elangiectasia occur. It is probably better not to distinguish such cases, as these

Characteristic findings and suggested treatment for limited cutaneous scleroderma		
Characteristic	Early stage	Late stage
Constitutional symptoms	• None	• Secondary to complications below
Skin thickening	• No or minimal progression	• Stable
Organs affected	• Raynaud's phenomenon, ulcers of digital tips, oesophageal symptoms	• Raynaud's phenomenon, ulcers of digital tips, calcinosis, oesophageal stricture, small bowel malabsorption, pulmonary hypertension
Treatment	• Vascular treatment (oral or intravenous) with or without digital sympathectomy, removal of calcinosis, treat oesophageal problems	• Vascular treatment (oral or intravenous) with or without digital sympathectomy, removal of calcinosis, treat oesophageal and midgut problems

Characteristic findings and suggested treatment for diffuse cutaneous scleroderma		
Characteristic	Early stage	Late stage
Constitutional symptoms	• Fatigue, weight loss	• None
Skin thickening	• Rapid progression	• Stable or regression
Organs affected	• Risk of renal, cardiac, pulmonary (fibrosis), gastrointestinal, articular, and muscular damage	• Musculoskeletal deformities, progression of existing visceral diseases but reduced risk of new complications
Treatment	• Immunosuppression, antifibrotic treatment, vasodilation, physiotherapy, and occupational therapy as appropriate	• Treat complications, reduce antifibrotic

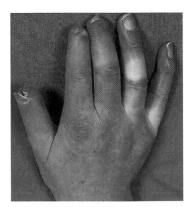 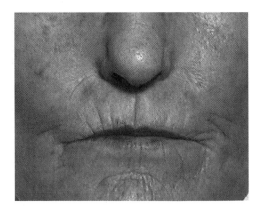 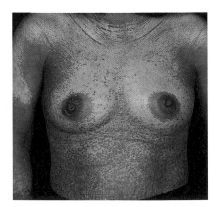

Characteristic features of limited cutaneous scleroderma. Left: Puffy fingers, tight skin, Raynaud's phenomenon, loss of distal digits, and ulceration of tips of digits. Middle: Microstomia and telangiectasia. Right: Hypopigmentation caused by diffuse cutaneous scleroderma

manifestations are not universal and underemphasise life-threatening complications that develop in a significant proportion of patients with limited cutaneous scleroderma. These include pulmonary arterial hypertension, severe midgut disease, and interstitial pulmonary fibrosis. Other cases of scleroderma include overlap syndromes with features of polyarthritis, myositis, or systemic lupus erythematosus, and the small group of scleroderma sine scleroderma with major visceral involvement, Raynaud's phenomenon, and hallmark autoantibodies (typically anti-topoisomerase 1). The term "mixed connective tissue disease" is probably best avoided, as most patients so designated develop a defined overlap syndrome, often with prominent features of scleroderma or lupus.

Autoantibody profiles

The major hallmark autoantibodies associated with scleroderma are mutually exclusive. If a patient has anticentromere antibodies, they almost never will have anti-topoisomerase 1 or another reactivity associated with scleroderma. This seems to reflect on the immunogenetic background of these patients and may explain clinical differences between patients with hallmark reactivity. Some antibodies, such as U1sn ribonucleotide protein, anti-Ku, and anti Th/To, are not exclusive, although they may identify patients with particular features.

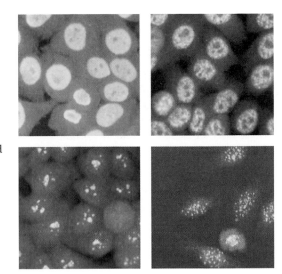

Common immunofluorescent patterns seen on testing for antinuclear antibodies. Top left: Homogeneous—typical of antibodies to DNA, with or without histones. Top right: Speckled—typical of antibodies to Ro, La, Sm, and ribonucleotide protein. Bottom left: Nucleolar—typical of scleroderma. Bottom right: Centromere—mainly found with limited cutaneous scleroderma

Autoimmune serology in scleroderma*

Antibody	Type of scleroderma	Prevalence (%)	Comments
ACA	Limited cutaneous scleroderma	60	• Associated with typical CREST
Scl-70	Diffuse cutaneous scleroderma	40	• Predictive of interstitial lung involvement, especially in limited cutaneous scleroderma
	Limited cutaneous scleroderma	15	
RNApol	Scleroderma	20	• Anti RNApol I or III associated with diffuse subset and renal disease
U1RNP	Scleroderma	10	• Associated with overlap features
U3RNP	Scleroderma	6	• Poor outcome and isolated pulmonary hypertension in diffuse cutaneous scleroderma
PM-Scl	Scleroderma	3	• Myositis overlap
Anti-M2 and M4	Scleroderma	10-15	• Especially in limited cutaneous scleroderma with primary biliary cirrhosis

*See also Chapters 18 and 20.

Risk stratification in scleroderma

The clinical heterogeneity of scleroderma, differences in the natural history of the two major subsets, and the life-threatening nature of some of the complications associated with scleroderma, have led to attempts to risk stratify patients at diagnosis and initial assessment. Abnormalities that reflect systemic inflammation (elevated erythrocyte sedimentation rate), pulmonary disease (impaired diffusing capacity for carbon monoxide), and renal involvement (proteinuria) identify patients with poor a prognosis at five years. The clinical association of antibody profiles also allows identification of patients at increased risk of pulmonary or renal complications. In the future, such information may direct management and screening. Genetic factors that determine the profile of the disease are being sought.

Management

Unfortunately, no disease modifying treatments are of proven efficacy currently. Most patients benefit from vascular therapy, and a number of agents that have the potential for vascular remodelling have been used in trials. Immunosuppressive

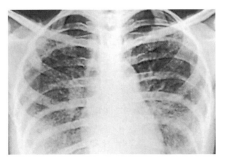

Chest radiograph of diffuse interstitial lung disease in a patient with scleroderma

Principles of management of systemic sclerosis

- Accurate diagnosis
- Appropriate allocation to a subset of scleroderma
- Stage the disease within the subset
- Consider disease modifying therapy
- Risk stratify for major organ based complications based upon serological, genetic, and clinical features
- Screen and start early intervention when complications develop
- Organ based therapy

treatment is generally reserved for patients with early and aggressive diffuse cutaneous scleroderma or with a major organ based complication, such as interstitial lung disease or myositis. A number of approaches are being evaluated in clinical trials, including oral tolerisation, type I bovine collagen, immunoablation, and autologous peripheral stem cell rescue. Currently, no antifibrotic agents are effective for established scleroderma, but a number are under development, including biological therapies that neutralise key potential cytokines that drive scleroderma (for example, transforming growth factor β1 and connective tissue growth factor).

Organ based complications

The outcome of scleroderma is determined largely by the extent and severity of organ based complications. Some of these are almost universal, such as oesophageal reflux, while many of the severe complications occur in around 10-15% of cases overall.

Pulmonary hypertension

Several major advances have been made in the field of pulmonary arterial hypertension that complicates scleroderma and other connective tissue diseases. Many of these are drawn from advances in the management of primary pulmonary arterial hypertension. Long-term warfarin should probably be given (with oesophagitis treatment) to all cases with definite pulmonary arterial hypertension. Prostanoids, in the form of prostacyclin analogues, seem to be effective. Iloprost or Epoprostenol are used currently and UT15 has recently also been licensed in the United States. Inhaled, intravenous, or subcutaneous administration have been shown to be superior to placebo in primary pulmonary arterial hypertension and by analogy are almost certainly effective in pulmonary arterial hypertension in patients with scleroderma. A particularly exciting development is the use of an orally active endothelin receptor blocker in pulmonary arterial hypertension. Raised endothelin-1 may be important in the pathogenesis of primary hypertension and the antagonist has beneficial effects on haemodynamic and exercise capacity in pulmonary arterial hypertension. Hopefully, additional therapies will soon become available. Transplantation is often difficult to obtain in patients with scleroderma with pulmonary arterial hypertension.

Lung fibrosis

This can occur in either of the two major subsets of scleroderma patients, although it is more common in diffuse cutaneous scleroderma. The anti-scl70 autoantibody provides a useful clinical marker and is generally associated with lung fibrosis in both subsets of scleroderma. Assessment of lung fibrosis has to be multidimensional. Interestingly, most cases of scleroderma have the histological pattern of non-specific interstitial pneumonia, whereas idiopathic disease is mostly of the usual interstitial pneumonia pattern. As the survival of patients matched for extent of disease is much worse in idiopathic disease, these histological differences may be very relevant. Interestingly, within the scleroderma subgroup, histological class does not seem to relate directly to outcome.

Scleroderma renal crisis

Major advances have been made in the management of renal disease in scleroderma. The major problems is one of recognition, so education of both patients and physicians is important. Scleroderma renal crisis often presents non-specifically with headaches and visual disturbances before

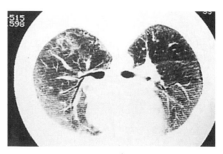

High resolution computed tomography scan showing evidence of early interstitial lung disease

encephalopathy, cardiac failure, or acute oliguric renal failure develop. Treatment with angiotensin converting enzyme inhibition is mandatory. Patients should be admitted for blood pressure control and monitoring of renal function. Generally, 50% of cases need dialysis, which is temporary in many patients. Significant recovery in renal function may be seen for up to two years after a renal crisis, and decisions regarding transplantation should be delayed until that time. Prophylactic angiotensin converting enzyme inhibition has contributed greatly to an improved outcome at all stages of renal disease in scleroderma.

Gut disease

The gastrointestinal tract is the most frequently affected organ in scleroderma. Up to 90% of patients have oesophageal dysmotility with reflux, and the proton pump inhibitors have dramatically improved symptomatic disease. Strictures are now relatively rare, although vigilance for Barrett's metaplasia is needed. Midgut disease with bacterial overgrowth may respond to broad spectrum antibiotics, although maintenance treatment may be required. Paradoxically, colonic involvement may lead to severe constipation and anorectal incontinence is prevalent. Acute abdominal complications of scleroderma must be managed conservatively wherever possible.

Further reading

- Denton CP, Black CM. Scleroderma and related disorders: therapeutic aspects. *Bailliére's Best Pract Res Clin Rheumatol* 2000;14:17-35
- Silver RM. Clinical aspects of systemic sclerosis (scleroderma). *Ann Rheum Dis* 1991;50:854-61
- LeRoy EC, Medsger TA Jr. Criteria for the classification of early systemic sclerosis. *J Rheumatol* 2001;28:1573-6
- Bouros D, Wells AU, Nicholson AG, Colby TV, Polychronopoulos V, Pantelidis P, et al. Histopathologic subsets of fibrosing alveolitis in patients with systemic sclerosis and their relationship to outcome. *Am J Respir Crit Care Med* 2002;165:1581-6
- Coghlan JG, Mukerjee D. The heart and pulmonary vasculature in scleroderma: clinical features and pathobiology. *Curr Opin Rheumatol* 2001;13:495-9
- Steen VD, Medsger TA Jr. Severe organ involvement in systemic sclerosis with diffuse scleroderma. *Arthritis Rheum* 2000;43: 2437-44

18   Is it a connective tissue disease?

Peter J Maddison

Clinical criteria to classify the major connective tissue diseases have been published (see Chapters 16 and 17). In each case, criteria were chosen because of their high sensitivity and specificity, but they were intended primarily as a means of standardising patient populations for clinical research rather than for diagnosis. They are extremely limited for early diagnosis of connective tissue diseases. The general experience of connective tissue disease clinics is that >50% of patients at a single point in time do not satisfy any criteria for connective tissue disease; although many patients eventually fulfil classification criteria for one of the major connective tissue disease entities, it may take 10-20 years.

Reasons for the continuing difficulty in diagnosing connective tissue diseases, even with modern laboratory aids, are various. In addition to the diverse clinical and laboratory features of the disease, a considerable number of patients present with non-specific symptoms: Raynaud's phenomenon, arthritis, fever, malaise, and fatigue. A substantial proportion of patients who present with a connective tissue disease also do not fit in the standard classification system. This has prompted the introduction of additional terms such as "overlap syndrome" and "undifferentiated connective tissue disease."

Diagnosis of connective tissue disease thus is still a great clinical challenge. Although patients with potentially aggressive disease must be recognised and treated appropriately at an early stage, patients with potentially benign disease must be recognised to avoid overtreatment.

Antinuclear antibodies in various diseases detected by indirect immunofluorescence

Condition	Frequency of antinuclear antibodies (%)
Autoimmune rheumatic disease	
• Drug induced lupus	100
• Systemic lupus erythematosus	98
• Systemic sclerosis	98
• Sjögren's syndrome	80
• Pauciarticular juvenile idiopathic arthritis	70
• Polymyositis or dermatomyositis	60
• Rheumatoid arthritis	50
Organ specific autoimmunity	
• Primary autoimmune cholangitis	100
• Autoimmune hepatitis	70
• Myasthenia gravis	50
• Autoimmune thyroid disease	45
Other conditions	
• Waldenstrom's macroglobulinaemia	20
• Subacute bacterial endocarditis	20
• Infectious mononucleosis	15
• Leprosy	15
Normal population	
• Children	8
• Adults	15

Specificity of antinuclear antibodies in diagnosis and disease expression

Disease	Antibody	Frequency (%)	Clinical association
Systemic lupus erythematosus	Anti-nDNA	70	• Lupus nephritis
	Anti-Sm	10-25*	• Vasculitis, central nervous system lupus
	Anti-U1RNP	30	• Raynaud's phenomenon, swollen fingers, arthritis, myositis, mixed connective tissue disease
	Anti-Ro	40	• Photosensitive rash, subacute cutaneous lupus erythematosus, neonatal lupus, congenital heart block, Sjögren's syndrome
	Anti-La	15	• As for anti-Ro
	Anti-rRNP	15	• Central nervous system lupus (psychosis or depression)
Sjögren's syndrome	Anti-Ro	60-90†	• Extraglandular disease, vasculitis, lymphoma
	Anti-La	35-85†	• As for anti-Ro
Systemic sclerosis	Anticentromere	30	• Limited cutaneous disease, microvascular or macrovascular disease, telangiectasia
	Anti-ThRNP	4	• Limited cutaneous disease
	Anti-topo-1	25	• Diffuse cutaneous disease, interstitial lung disease
	Anti-RNA polymerases	20	• Diffuse cutaneous disease, renal disease
	Anti-U3RNP	5	• Diffuse cutaneous disease, pulmonary hypertension
	Anti-PM-Scl	5	• Scleroderma or polymyositis overlap
	Anti-Ku	2	• Scleroderma or polymyositis overlap
Dermatomyositis and polymyositis	Anti-Jo-1	30	• Antisynthetase syndrome (antisynthetase syndrome)
	(antibodies to other tRNA synthetases)	(3)	
	Anti-SRP	4	• Severe myositis
	Anti-Mi2	10	• Dermatomyositis

*Higher frequency in people of African or Indian origin. †With sensitive enzyme linked immunosorbent assays.

Autoantibody profile in diagnosis

Antinuclear antibodies are a hallmark of connective tissue diseases. Serology is of particular value in situations where clinical expression of the disease is incomplete, when the presence of a particular antinuclear antibody profile can be diagnostic. They can be found in a variety of clinical settings, however, and their occurrence does not necessarily indicate the presence of any disease. It is imperative therefore that tests for antinuclear antibodies are requested and that the results are interpreted in the light of the clinical findings.

Certain autoantibody profiles are associated with diagnostic categories of connective tissue disease and sometimes with particular patterns of clinical manifestations. These autoantibodies are usually present from the beginning of the clinical presentation and are detectable throughout the course of the disease. Once antinuclear antibodies have been detected with a screening test, therefore, it is important to determine their specificity. This is now part of the standard operating procedure of serology laboratories, but the process is greatly facilitated by the doctor giving enough clinical information when antinuclear antibodies testing is requested.

The HEp2 cell substrate enhances the sensitivity of the test for antinuclear antibodies in systemic lupus erythematosus, so that antinuclear antibodies can be detected in 95% of untreated patients with active disease. When a doctor wants to exclude systemic lupus erythematosus, immunofluorescence is enough as a screening test for antinuclear antibodies, and it is not cost-effective to test automatically for anti-DNA or other antibody specificities. In some instances, the immunofluorescence test for antinuclear antibodies gives a false negative result; this may occur if the antigen is outside the nucleus (for example, anti-Jo-1 and anti-ribosomal P, both often categorised under the umbrella term "antinuclear antibodies") or if it is present in a form not recognised by a particular autoantibody (for example, when anti-Ro is directed exclusively to determinants on the native Ro molecule not expressed in cultured HEp-2 cells). In such cases, the clinical picture dictates that specific assays should be undertaken.

Undifferentiated connective tissue disease

The term "undifferentiated connective tissue disease" was first coined in 1980 by LeRoy and colleagues to counter the concept of mixed connective tissue disease being a distinct disease entity and to point out that many patients designated as having mixed connective tissue disease presented with an early phase of disease that later evolved into one of the "classic" connective tissue diseases, particularly scleroderma. Subsequently, undifferentiated connective tissue disease has been embraced by others and, rather than replacing mixed connective tissue disease, it has been used to describe patients with clinical and laboratory features of connective tissue disease that do not fulfil criteria for any one disorder. Although no universally agreed definition of "undifferentiated connective tissue disease" exists, this term should be distinguished from other commonly used terms such as "overlap syndrome," in which patients meet the criteria for two or more connective tissue disease or specific criteria for mixed connective tissue disease (see also Chapters 16 and 17). Other terms used in the literature that are synonymous with undifferentiated connective tissue disease include "pre-lupus," "latent lupus," or "incomplete lupus."

Long-term, prospective follow up studies of outcome show that these patients represent a large proportion

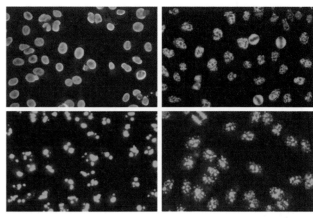

Individual antinuclear antibody fluorescent patterns are of limited diagnostic utility but may provide guidance to more specific immunological tests

Terminology

Undifferentiated connective tissue disease	• Patient has features seen in connective tissue disease but does not meet criteria for a defined connective tissue disease
Overlap	• Patients meet criteria for two or more connective tissue diseases
Mixed connective tissue disease	• Overlap with rheumatoid arthritis-like arthritis, systemic lupus erythematosus, scleroderma, and myositis with antibodies to U1RNP

Characteristics of undifferentiated connective tissue disease

- Comprise a large proportion (20-50%) of referrals for connective tissue disease
- Common manifestations
  Raynaud's
  Arthralgia or myalgia
  Rash
  Sicca symptoms
- Some (20-50%) evolve into a defined connective tissue disease, usually within two years

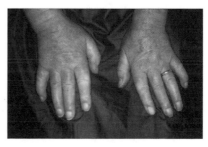

Swollen fingers of patient with undifferentiated connective tissue disease

(20-50%, depending on the study) of patients presenting with connective tissue diseases. The most common clinical features are Raynaud's phenomenon, polyarthritis, mucocutaneous manifestations, non-specific features such as fatigue, and positive antinuclear antibodies. The major organ systems are involved only rarely. Although the disease evolves to fulfil classification criteria of a defined connective tissue disease in a minority of patients (about 30% in the larger studies), other outcomes include spontaneous remission and the persistence of the undifferentiated connective tissue disease state, which is the most usual outcome. Evolution to a "full blown" connective tissue disease, if it happens, usually occurs in the first few years of follow up, generally within two years of presentation.

Differential diagnosis of connective tissue diseases

A common clinical conundrum is the distinction of systemic lupus erythematosus from other connective tissue diseases. All frequently present with a mixture of systemic symptoms, including fever and weight loss, and musculoskeletal and/or mucocutaneous involvement. The combination of a careful history and physical examination, urine analysis, chest x ray, laboratory tests for an acute phase response, blood count, serum biochemistry, complement levels, creatine kinase, and serological profile, however, results in the correct diagnosis in a high proportion of cases.

Drug induced lupus
A carefully elicited drug history is essential to exclude drug induced lupus. The management of this is very straightforward, involving discontinuation of the offending agent and short-term anti-inflammatory treatment. Procainamide and hydralazine carry the highest risk of inducing a lupus-like syndrome. These are now prescribed infrequently, but many drugs are still associated with well documented drug induced lupus. The clinical presentation is similar to that of idiopathic systemic lupus erythematosus, with systemic features including fever and weight loss, arthralgia or frank arthritis, and serositis (particularly common with procainamide). Major organ involvement, such as nephritis and central nervous system manifestations, is less common. A high level of antinuclear antibodies usually shows a homogeneous pattern from the earliest presentation, and the typical preponderance of anti-histone antibodies can be shown with specific assays. Antibodies to native DNA and "extractable nuclear antigens," commonly associated with idiopathic systemic lupus erythematosus, are almost invariably negative. The gold standard for diagnosis of drug induced lupus, however, is that it resolves after the drug is stopped; the symptoms improve within days to weeks, although the antinuclear antibodies may take a year or two to disappear.

In two drug induced lupus syndromes diagnosis is often difficult or overlooked. The first is associated with minocycline. Although the risk of this complication is low, the drug is prescribed often for acne, and many cases have now been reported. Often, the affected individual does not consider their "acne remedy" to be a drug and specific enquiry about minocycline needs to be made. The second example is associated with sulfasalazine, which is often used as a disease modifying antirheumatic drug in rheumatoid arthritis. Again, this drug carries a low risk of inducing lupus. Sometimes, the diagnosis is difficult to make in the context of rheumatoid arthritis, particularly as antinuclear antibodies are present in about 50% of patients with the condition. Renal disease can

Distinguishing features of connective tissue diseases	
Condition	**Distinguishing features**
Systemic rheumatic diseases	
• Rheumatoid arthritis	• Prominent signs of synovitis; multisystem involvement uncommon at presentation; no autoantibodies associated with connective tissue disease
• Systemic sclerosis	• Pronounced Raynaud's phenomenon; scleroderma; characteristic serological profile
• Dermatomyositis	• Distinctive pattern of eruption; prominent muscle involvement; serological profile
• Primary vasculitis	• Distinctive renal involvement; neutrophilia (sometimes eosinophilia); serological profile
• Behçet's syndrome	• Lack of typical serological features
• Adult Still's disease	• Typical fever pattern; lack of typical serological features
• Periodic fever syndromes (familial Mediterranean fever, tumour necrosis factor associated periodic syndrome, hyperimmunoglobulin D, etc)	• Intermittent manifestations; no autoantibodies associated with connective tissue disease
Other systemic disorders	
• Autoimmune hepatitis	• Typical liver involvement; absence of typical lupus features
• Sarcoidosis	• Typical histology; no autoantibodies associated with connective tissue disease
• Angioimmunoblastic lymphadenopathy	• Typical histology; no autoantibodies associated with connective tissue disease
Other causes of photosensitivity and red face	
• Polymorphous light eruption	• Lack of systemic features; different histology; absent autoantibodies
• Rosacea	• Papulopustular eruption; non-systemic; absent autoantibodies
• Seborrhoeic dermatitis	• Different morphology and histology; non-systemic, absent autoantibodies
• Contact dermatitis	• History of allergen contact; pseudovesicle; no autoantibodies
• Jessner's benign lymphocytic infiltration	• Typical histology; negative serology
• Erythrohepatic protoporphyria	• Vesicobullous lesions; urinary and plasma porphyrin profile; no antibodies associated with systemic lupus erythematosus
• Syphilis	• Typical histology; diagnostic serology
Other causes of fatigue and musculoskeletal pain	
• Fibromyalgia	• No objective inflammation; no autoantibodies associated with connective tissue disease

Features of drug induced lupus
- History of exposure to relevant drug
- Renal and central nervous system manifestations rare
- Antinuclear antibodies directed primarily to histones
- Features resolve on discontinuing drug

occur in sulfasalazine induced lupus, however, particularly in those in whom the diagnosis has been overlooked.

Which connective tissue disease?

Although the clinical presentation in the early stage can be similar between connective tissue diseases, the evolution of typical clinical features over weeks or months is usually enough to distinguish the characteristic patterns associated with the different diseases. Early diagnosis is aided by recognition of distinctive serological profiles that are generally present with the earliest clinical manifestations. Diagnosis can also be facilitated by typical laboratory abnormalities and histological changes in the tissues involved. For example, microscopic polyangiitis that presents with weight loss, fever, polyarthritis, and active urinary sediment can be distinguished from lupus by an autoimmune response primarily to myeloperoxidase and the typical histological picture of pauci-immune focal necrotising glomerulonephritis. Similarly, dermatomyositis sine myositis that presents with photosensitive eruptions on the face, arms, and hands and is associated with myalgia can be distinguished from lupus by the distribution of the eruption, a raised serum creatine kinase, and typical changes on muscle biopsy, despite the absence of frank weakness.

Diagnosis is often complicated if lupus is part of an overlap syndrome and the patient fulfils classification criteria of more than one connective tissue disease (as opposed to undifferentiated connective tissue disease). The most common overlaps with systemic lupus erythematosus are patients who also have features of systemic sclerosis, polymyositis, or both, and patients with rheumatoid arthritis. Sometimes patients present with an overlap syndrome; at other times, the picture evolves sequentially. Development of Sjögren's syndrome during the course of systemic lupus erythematosus is well established, but, occasionally, patients with primary Sjögren's syndrome develop typical features of lupus, especially photosensitive eruptions typical of subacute cutaneous lupus erythematosus, after many years of disease.

Patients with an overlap of systemic lupus erythematosus and scleroderma or polymyositis, or both, often have a distinctive serological profile that includes high levels of antibodies to U1RNP. These patients have been suggested to have a distinctive connective tissue disease "mixed connective tissue disease." This concept is very controversial, however, with critics and protagonists (see also Chapters 16 and 17).

A number of series report patients who fulfil criteria for both systemic lupus erythematosus and rheumatoid arthritis. For these patients, the term "rhupus" has been coined. These patients are usually easier to recognise when the rheumatoid arthritis develops first, but they are characterised ultimately by typical rheumatoid features such as erosive arthritis, subcutaneous nodules, and rheumatoid factor. These features are accompanied by cutaneous, renal, haematological, and other clinical manifestations characteristic of systemic lupus erythematosus but unusual for rheumatoid arthritis, with the presence of autoantibodies to nDNA.

Features that suggest underlying connective tissue disease

- Onset in early childhood or later adult life
- Asymmetrical involvement of fingers
- Evidence of digital ischaemic damage
- Abnormal morphology of nailfold capillaries (including dilated, distorted capillaries and areas of capillary dropout)
- Presence of autoantibodies associated with connective tissue disease

---

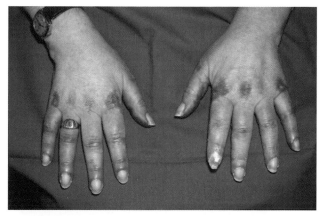

Hands in systemic lupus erythemataosus

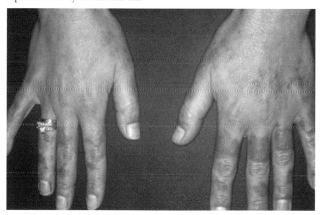

Finger pulp scars from previous digital ischaemic ulceration in a patient with systemic sclerosis

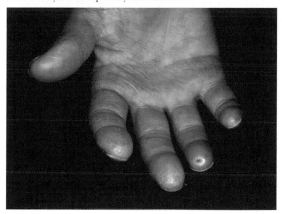

Hands in dermatomyositis

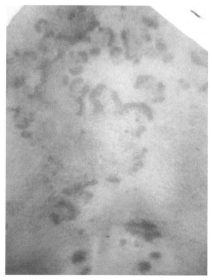

Rash in subacute cutaneous lupus erythematosus

Raynaud's phenomenon

Raynaud's phenomenon is often the presenting manifestation of connective tissue diseases, especially systemic sclerosis. It is common, however, in otherwise healthy people.

Other disorders of the skin

One of the most common conundrums that I meet in my lupus clinic is the patient referred with a history of photosensitivity or red face in association with musculoskeletal symptoms and, perhaps, systemic features such as fatigue. Photosensitive eruptions are common in the normal female population or may be induced by, for example, non-steroidal anti-inflammatory drugs. About 10% of women develop polymorphous light eruption—a pruritic papular eruption that occurs within hours of sun exposure, typically on normally covered sites, that spares the face and hands, and that resolves within days without epidermal change. In contrast, photosensitivity in systemic lupus erythematosus also affects face and hands. The latent period after sun exposure is usually longer, the skin is less pruritic, and the eruption persists longer.

Similarly, although facial erythema is seen typically in patients with systemic lupus erythematosus, it must be distinguished from other causes. Typical rosaceae consists of papulopustular lesions on a background of telangiectasia. Sometimes, light exposure aggravates this condition and a biopsy is sometimes needed to distinguish atypical forms from lupus. Benign lymphocytic infiltration, such as Jessner's, may produce papular or annular lesions that are indistinguishable clinically from subacute cutaneous lupus erythematosus and papular lupus erythematosus. The typical histological appearance includes a dense dermal lymphocytic infiltrate without the characteristic epidermal changes of lupus. Seborrhoeic dermatitis may affect the cheeks and paranasal folds and is usually pruritic and associated with desquamation. Contact dermatitis, which may be caused by cosmetics, produces superficial erythema, pseudovesicles, and sometimes eyelid swelling.

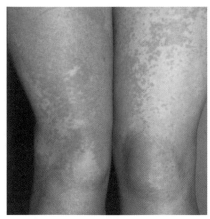
Polymorphous light eruption

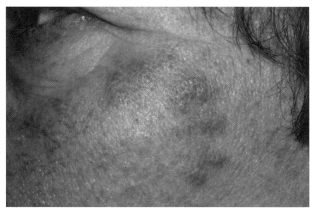
Papular light eruption and Jessner's

Fibromyalgia

Fibromyalgia syndrome (see Chapter 7) is often mistaken for lupus, especially if the test for antinuclear antibodies is also positive, and sometimes is treated inappropriately with, for example, corticosteroids. In addition, a significant proportion of people with fibromyalgia have other features that could be interpreted as manifestations of a connective tissue disease such as Raynaud's phenomenon, sicca symptoms, and cognitive dysfunction. In those mistakenly treated with corticosteroids, although no evidence shows therapeutic efficacy in fibromyalgia, steroid withdrawal can make the symptoms worse. No evidence exists of an increased prevalence of positive antinuclear antibodies or the occurrence of connective tissue disease in patients with fibromyalgia. It has become increasingly apparent, however, that patients with connective tissue disease—especially those with systemic lupus erythematosus and Sjögren's syndrome—have a high prevalence of fibromyalgia that makes a considerable contribution to morbidity but is unrelated to the activity of the disease.

Is it infection?

Some infections can mimic connective tissue disease, especially systemic lupus erythematosus; these include HIV, syphilis, tuberculosis, and persistent infections with viruses such as Epstein-Barr virus and cytomegalovirus. They can present with

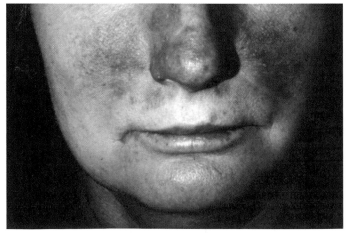
Rosaceae papules and pustules

mucocutaneous manifestations, fever, malaise, polyarthralgia, lymphadenopathy, and serological abnormalities, such as positive tests for antinuclear antibodies and rheumatoid factor.

A more commonly encountered clinical conundrum is how to distinguish infection from a flare up of disease in a patient with systemic lupus erythematosus. Bacterial infections occur more commonly in lupus patients than in matched controls. Even patients in remission have an increased risk of infection, and this is enhanced by corticosteroid treatment. Infections generally involve the commonly occurring pyogenic organisms such as *Staphylococcus* species and *Escherichia coli*, but opportunistic infections also occur, especially in patients who take high dose corticosteroids and immunosuppressive agents.

Measurement of C reactive protein has been suggested as a way of distinguishing between infection and active lupus. Most studies have reported generally higher levels of C reactive protein in patients with infection compared with those with active disease; the proposal was that levels of C reactive protein >60 mg/l strongly indicated infection and with levels of C reactive protein < 30 mg/l infection was very unlikely. High levels of C reactive protein can be seen in patients without infection but with a lupus flare that particularly involves the joints and serositis, however, and levels of C reactive protein have been shown to be an unreliable predictor of infection in prospective longitudinal studies.

In the absence of useful surrogate markers of infection in systemic lupus erythematosus, exhaustive microbiological investigations and early and often repeated cultures, sometimes from affected tissues, are needed to make a definitive diagnosis.

Further reading

- Benedek TG. Historical background of discoid and systemic lupus erythematosus. In: Wallace DJ, Hahn BH, eds. *Duboisâ lupus erythematosus.* 5th ed. Baltimore: Williams and Wilkins, 1997, pp. 3-16
- Liang MH, Meenan RF, Cathcart ES, Schur PH. A screening strategy for population studies in systemic lupus erythematosus: series design. *Arthritis Rheum* 1980;23:152-7
- Alarcon GS. Unclassified or undifferentiated connective tissue disease. *Baillière's Best Pract Res Clin Rheumatol* 2000;14:125-37
- Swaak AJG, van de Brink H, Smeenk RJT, Manger K, Kalden JR, Tosi S, et al. Incomplete lupus erythematosus: results of a multicentre study under the supervision of the EULAR Standing Committee on International Clinical Studies Including Therapeutic Trials (ESCISIT). *Rheumatology* 2001;40:89-94
- Lawson TM, Amos N, Bulgen D, Williams BD. Minocycline-induced lupus: clinical features and response to rechallenge. *Rheumatology* 2001;40:329-35
- Gunnarsson I, Kanerud L, Pettersson E, Lundberg I, Lindblad S, Ringertz B. Predisposing factors in sulphasalazine-induced systemic lupus erythematosus. *Br J Rheumatol* 1997;36:1089-94
- Maddison PJ. MCTD: overlap syndromes. *Baillière's Best Pract Res Clin Rheumatol* 2000;14:111-24
- Bennett R. The concurrence of lupus and fibromyalgia: implications for diagnosis and management. *Lupus* 1997;6: 494-9
- Fessler BJ. Infectious diseases in systemic lupus erythematosus: risk factors, management and prophylaxis. *Baillière's Best Pract Res Clin Rheumatol* 2002;16:281-91
- Isenberg DA, Ehrenstein MR. Systemic Lupus Erythematosus. In: Isenberg DA, Maddison PJ, Woo P, Glass DN, Breedveld F, eds. *Oxford textbook of rheumatology.* 3rd ed. Oxford: Oxford Medical Publications, 2003

19   Vasculitis and related rashes

Richard A Watts, David GI Scott

The vasculitides are a heterogeneous group of uncommon diseases characterised by inflammatory cell infiltration and necrosis of blood vessel walls. Systemic necrotising vasculitis can be rapidly life-threatening, so early accurate diagnosis and treatment is vital. Vasculitis may be primary (Wegener's granulomatosis, Churg-Strauss syndrome, microscopic polyangiitis, and polyarteritis nodosa) or secondary to established connective tissue disease (such as rheumatoid arthritis), infection, or malignancy. The severity of vasculitis is related to the size and site of the vessels affected. Classification is based on vessel size and determines the treatment approach.

Large vessel vasculitis

Large vessel vasculitis includes giant cell arteritis and Takayasu's arteritis. Giant cell arteritis is described elsewhere (Chapter 15). Takayasu's arteritis is uncommon and affects young adults, who initially present with a non-specific illness and later with loss of pulses, claudication (especially of the upper limbs), and stroke.

Medium vessel vasculitis

Classical polyarteritis nodosa—A multisystem vasculitis characterised by formation of aneurysms in medium sized arteries. Patients present with a constitutional illness, which is often associated with rash, mononeuritis multiplex, vascular hypertension, and organ infarction. Polyarteritis nodosa may be confined to the skin. Angiography shows typical aneurysms. Polyarteritis nodosa has been associated with chronic hepatitis B antigenaemia.

Kawasaki disease (mucocutaneous lymph node syndrome)—An acute vasculitis that primarily affects infants and young children. It presents with fever, rash, lymphadenopathy, and palmoplantar erythema. Coronary arteries become affected in up to one quarter of untreated patients; this can lead to myocardial ischaemia and infarction.

Medium and small vessel vasculitis

This group includes the major necrotising vasculitides: microscopic polyangiitis, Wegener's granulomatosis, and Churg-Strauss syndrome, with involvement of both medium and small arteries. These may occur at any age, with the peak incidence at 60-70 years. Primary systemic vasculitis is slightly more common in men. The annual incidence is about 20 cases per million people. The symptoms depend on the size and site of vessel affected and on the individual diagnosis.

Wegener's granulomatosis—This is characterised by a granulomatous vasculitis of the upper and lower respiratory tracts and glomerulonephritis, but almost any organ system can be affected. The lungs are affected in 45% of patients at diagnosis. Symptoms in the ear, nose, and throat (such as epistaxis, crusting, and deafness) particularly are associated with this condition, and they should be sought in all patients with suspected vasculitis. Patients with limited Wegener's granulomatosis—disease without renal involvement—may have a better prognosis. Biopsy of affected organs shows a necrotising arteritis, often with formation of granulomas.

Classification of vasculitis

Vessels predominantly affected	Primary	Secondary
• Larger arteries	• Giant cell arteritis • Takayasu's arteritis	• Aortitis associated with rheumatoid arthritis • Infection (syphilis)
• Medium arteries	• Classic polyarteritis nodosa • Kawasaki disease	• Infection (such as hepatitis B)
• Medium arteries and small vessels	• Wegener's granulomatosis* • Churg-Strauss syndrome • Microscopic polyangiitis	• Rheumatoid arthritis, systemic lupus erythematosus • Sjögren's syndrome • Drugs • Infection (HIV)
• Small vessels (leucocytoclastic)	• Henoch-Schönlein purpura • Cryoglobulinaemia leucocytoclastic vasculitis	• Drugs (such as sulphonamides, penicillins, thiazide diuretics, etc) • Infection

Symptoms suggestive of vasculitis

Systemic
- Malaise
- Fever
- Weight loss
- Myalgia
- Arthralgia

Skin
- Purpura (palpable)
- Ulceration
- Infarction

Gastrointestinal
- Mouth ulcers
- Abdominal pain
- Diarrhoea

Respiratory
- Cough
- Wheeze
- Haemoptysis
- Dyspnoea

Ear, nose, and throat
- Epistaxis
- Crusting
- Sinusitis
- Deafness

Cardiac
- Chest pain

Neurological
- Sensory or motor impairment

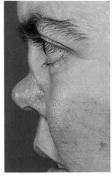 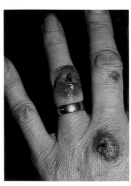

Wegener's granulomatosis. Left: Typical saddle nose deformity (reproduced with patient's permission). Right: Vasculitic rash

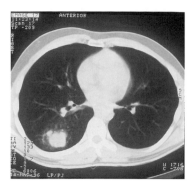

Computed tomography scan of thorax showing a granuloma in Wegener's granulomatosis

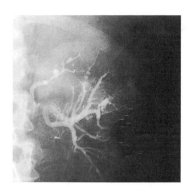

Coeliac axis arteriogram showing typical aneurysm in polyarteritis nodosa

Microscopic polyangiitis—This is characterised by vasculitis that affects the kidneys and sometimes the lungs.

Biopsy of the kidney shows a focal segmental necrotising glomerulonephritis with few immune deposits (sometimes called pauci immune vasculitis). Lung involvement usually presents with haemoptysis caused by pulmonary capillaritis and haemorrhage (pulmonary–renal syndrome).

Churg-Strauss syndrome—This syndrome is characterised by atopy (especially late onset asthma), pulmonary involvement (75% of patients have radiographic evidence of infiltration), and eosinophilia ($>1 \times 10^9/l$) in the tissues and peripheral blood. Such features can develop several years before the onset of systemic vasculitis. Cardiac involvement is a particular feature of Churg-Strauss syndrome and determines prognosis. Neuropathy is common.

Small vessel vasculitis

Small vessel vasculitis (leucocytoclastic or hypersensitivity) is usually confined to the skin, but it may be part of a systemic illness. The rash is purpuric, sometimes palpable, and occurs in dependent areas. The lesions may become bullous and ulcerate. Nailfold infarcts occur. Biopsy shows a cellular infiltrate of small vessels often with leucocytoclasis (fragmented polymorphonuclear cells and nuclear dust). Small vessel vasculitis has number of causes; drugs and infection are the most common.

Henoch-Schönlein purpura—This is a form of small vessel vasculitis that occurs mainly in childhood and young adults. Patients present with rash, arthritis, abdominal pain, and sometimes renal involvement. Deposits of immunoglobulin A can be detected histologically in the skin and renal mesangium.

Cryoglobulinaemia—Cryoglobulins are plasma proteins that precipitate in the cold. The condition presents with rash (including purpura digital ischaemia and ulcers), arthralgias, and neuropathy. A strong link exists between infection with hepatitis C virus and essential mixed cryoglobulinaemia: 80-90% of such patients are positive for anti-hepatitis C virus antibodies.

Investigation of vasculitis

Assessing inflammation
- Blood count and differential (total white cell count, eosinophils)
- Acute phase response (erythrocyte sedimentation rate, C reactive protein)
- Liver function

Assessment of organ involvement
- Urine analysis (proteinuria, haematuria, protein excretion, biopsy)
- Renal function (creatinine clearance, 24-hour protein excretion, biopsy)
- Chest radiograph
- Liver function
- Nervous system (nerve conduction studies, biopsy)
- Cardiac function (electrocardiograph, echocardiography)
- Gut (angiography)

Immunological tests
- Antineutrophil cytoplasmic antibodies (including proteinase 3 and myeloperoxidase antibodies)
- Other autoantibodies (rheumatoid factor, antinuclear antibodies, anticardiolipin antibodies)
- Complement
- Cryoglobulins

Differential diagnosis
- Blood cultures
- Viral serology
- Echocardiography

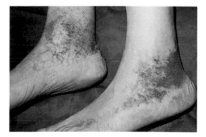

Vasculitic rash in cryoglobulinaemia

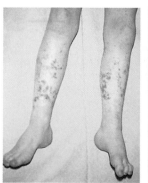
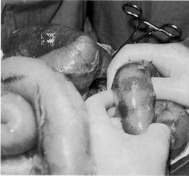

Small vessel vasculitis in Henoch-Schönlein purpura. Left: Affecting the skin. Right: Affecting the gut

---

Important mimics of vasculitis

- Subacute bacterial endocarditis
- Atrial myxoma
- Cholesterol embolism
- Antiphospholipid antibody syndrome

Differential diagnosis of rash and arthritis

- Infection
- Drug reaction
- Sarcoidosis
- Juvenile chronic arthritis
- Connective tissue disease
- Psoriasis
- Vasculitis

Investigation

Investigation aims to establish and confirm the diagnosis, the extent and severity of organ involvement, and disease activity.

Urine analysis—This is the most important investigation because the extent of renal involvement is one of the key determinants of prognosis. Detection of proteinuria or haematuria in a patient with systemic illness needs immediate further investigation and the patient is a medical emergency.

Blood tests—Leucocytosis suggests a primary vasculitis or infection. Leucopenia is associated with vasculitis secondary to a connective tissue disease (typically systemic lupus erythematosus). Eosinophilia suggests Churg-Strauss syndrome or a drug reaction.

Liver function tests—Abnormal results suggest viral infection (hepatitis A, B, or C) or may be non-specific.

Immunology—Antineutrophil cytoplasmic antibodies are associated with the primary systemic necrotising vasculitides (see Chapter 20). Cytoplasmic antineutrophil cytoplasmic antibodies in association with proteinase 3 antibodies are highly specific (>90%) for Wegener's granulomatosis. Perinuclear antineutrophil cytoplasmic antibodies associated with myeloperoxidase antibodies typically are found in microscopic polyangiitis and Churg-Strauss syndrome. Rheumatoid factors and antinuclear antibodies may indicate vasculitis associated with connective tissue disease. Complement levels are low in infection and lupus but high in primary vasculitis.

Biopsy—Tissue biopsy is important to confirm the diagnosis before treatment with potentially toxic immunosuppressive drugs. The choice of tissue to biopsy is crucial.

Other investigations—Angiography can show aneurysms. Blood cultures, viral serology, and echocardiography are important to exclude infection and other conditions that may present as systemic multisystem disease and mimic vasculitis.

Differential diagnosis

Livedo reticularis
Livedo reticularis is characterised by persistent patchy reddish-blue mottling of the legs (and occasionally arms) that is exacerbated by cold weather. It may lead to ulceration and is associated with vascular thrombosis (Sneddon's syndrome) and the presence of antiphospholipid antibodies. It is also a feature of polyarteritis nodosa and cryoglobulinaemia.

Bacterial infections
Direct bacterial infection of small arteries and arterioles infection causes a necrotising vasculitis or thrombosis. *Neisseria gonorrhoeae*, *N meningitides*, and *Streptobacillus moniliformis*, for example, may infect the vascular endothelium directly and cause maculopapular or purpuric skin lesions. Biopsies of early lesions show small vessel vasculitis. The organisms can be cultured from an aspirate of the lesions.

Infective endocarditis
Several organisms—streptococci, staphylococci, Gram negative bacilli, and *Coxiella*—can cause endocarditis. Polyarthritis may be accompanied by splinter haemorrhages, Janeway lesions

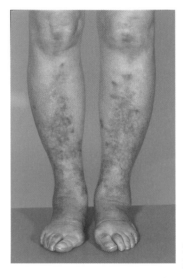

Livedo rash in cutaneous polyarteritis nodosa

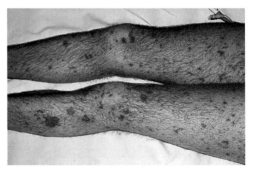

Haemorrhagic pustular rash in disseminated infection with *Neisseria meningitides*

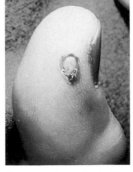
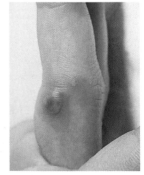

Gonococcal pustules in disseminated infection with *Neisseria gonorrhoeae*

(red macules over thenar and hypothenar eminences), Osler's nodes (tender papules over extremities of fingers and toes), and clubbing. Diagnosis is by blood culture and echocardiography.

Cholesterol embolism

Cholesterol embolism may occur spontaneously or after trauma to the aortic wall during vascular surgery or angiographic procedures. Typical cutaneous manifestations are ischaemia of the digits, particularly the toes from abdominal atheroma, emboli, and livedo reticularis that affects the legs. The ischaemic toe usually presents as sudden onset of a small, cool, cyanotic and painful area of the foot (usually the toe). The lesions are tender to touch and may progress to ulceration, digital infarction, and gangrene; this mimics systemic vasculitis. Presentation may be with a systemic illness caused by tissue inflammation; features include eosinophilia and a positive test for antineutrophil cytoplasmic antibodies.

Atrial myxoma

Cardiac myxomata are rare benign tumours found most often in the left atrium (90% of cases). Constitutional symptoms and systemic embolisation may lead to a wrong diagnosis of vasculitis. Systemic manifestations seen in 90% of cases include fever, weight loss, Raynaud's phenomenon, clubbing, elevated acute phase proteins, and hypergammaglobulinaemia. It is treated by surgical resection of the primary tumour and emboli.

Antiphospholipid antibody syndrome

Antiphospholipid antibody syndrome may present as catastrophic widespread thrombosis, and this can mimic systemic vasculitis. Livedo reticularis is the most typical cutaneous lesion and it occurs in association with thrombosis and recurrent fetal loss.

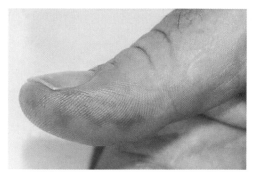

Janeway lesions in infective endocarditis

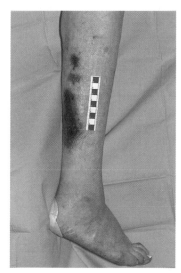

Cholesterol emboli

Prognosis

The natural history of untreated primary systemic vasculitis is of a rapidly progressive, usually fatal disease. Before corticosteroids were introduced in Wegener's granulomatosis, the median survival was five months, with 82% of patients dying within one year and more than 90% within two years. The introduction of corticosteroids improved survival in polyarteritis nodosa to 50% at five years. The median survival in Wegener's granulomatosis, was only 12.5 months using corticosteroids alone, with most patients dying of sepsis or uncontrolled disease. The introduction of oral low dose cyclophosphamide combined with prednisolone resulted in a significant improvement in the mortality of Wegener's granulomatosis, with a survival rate at five years of 82%.

Small vessel vasculitis confined to the skin without necrotising features has an excellent prognosis. Large vessel vasculitis has a good prognosis.

Treatment

Randomised controlled trials to inform and guide therapy of vasculitis generally are lacking. Treatment depends on the size of vessel involved. Small vessel vasculitis can often be treated conservatively, and large vessel vasculitis responds well to corticosteroids (oral prednisolone 40-60 mg/day), but treatment is usually needed for more than one year. The dose of corticosteroid should be reduced rapidly according to

---

Aims of management of vasculitis

- Induction of remission
- Maintenance of remission
- Recognition and early treatment of relapse
- Avoidance of drug toxicity

Treatment regimens for cyclophosphamide

Continuous low oral dose

Cyclophosphamide	2 mg/kg/day
Prednisolone	1 mg/kg/day

Oral pulse

Cyclophosphamide	5 mg/kg/day for three days
Prednisolone	1 mg/kg/day for three days

Intravenous pulse*

Cyclophosphamide	10-15 mg/kg[†]
Prednisolone	1 g

Cyclophopshamide dose should be adjusted according to white cell count, renal function, and clinical response.
*Pulse frequency: fortnightly (×6), every three weeks (×2), monthly (×6). Adjusted according to clinical response and toxicity.
[†] White cell count should be checked 7, 10, and 14 days after the first two pulses and immediately before subsequent pulses.

clinical and laboratory parameters, with the aim of reducing the dose to ≤10 mg within six months.

The introduction of cyclophosphamide combined with corticosteroids dramatically improved the prognosis of systemic necrotising vasculitis. Cyclophosphamide can be given either as continuous low dose oral therapy or intermittent pulse therapy. Both routes are equally effective at inducing remission, but pulse therapy is probably associated with a slightly higher relapse rate. The major toxicities of cyclophosphamide are haemorrhagic cystitis, formation of bladder tumours, infertility, and infection. Toxicity depends on the cumulative dose, so pulse therapy is less toxic. Mesna may reduce the frequency of bladder toxicity with intravenous cyclophosphamide. Fertile males should be offered sperm storage before they are given cyclophosphamide; ovarian function is less severely affected by pulse regimens. Prophylaxis with trimethoprim-sulfamethoxazole should be considered to prevent infection with *Pneumocystis carinii*.

Corticosteroids are started at a dose of 1 mg/kg and the dose is reduced quite rapidly so that the drug can be discontinued at around 12 months. Alternate day dosing may reduce the risk of infection.

The current trend is for shorter duration of cyclophosphamide therapy to reduce overall toxicity. Once remission has been achieved with cyclophosphamide (usually after 3-6 months) azathioprine is substituted. Cyclophosphamide should not be continued for more than one year because of the risks of toxicity. Weekly oral methotrexate is a possible alternative to azathioprine for maintenance therapy. Survival has improved and remission can be obtained in most patients, but many need prolonged immunosuppressive therapy (5-10 years), and the rate of relapse is still substantial (50% at five years).

Plasmapheresis is reserved for patients with pulmonary haemorrhage and severe renal disease. Intravenous immunoglobulin is effective in the treatment of Kawasaki disease, but its role in other vasculitides, where it induces temporary improvement, is uncertain at present. The role of tumour necrosis factor α blocking drugs and mycophenolate mofetil is being explored.

Further reading

- Ball GV, Bridges L, eds. *Vasculitis*. Oxford: Oxford University Press, 2002
- Jayne D. Update on the European Vasculitis Study Group trials. *Curr Opin Rheumatol* 1999;13:48-55
- Jayne D. Evidence based treatment of systemic vasculitis. *Rheumatology* 2000;39:585-95
- Langford C. Treatment of polyarteritis nodosa, Microscopic polyangiitis, and Churg-Strauss syndrome: where do we stand now? *Arthritis Rheum* 2001;44:508-12
- Langford C, Talar-Williams C, Barron K, Sneller M. A staged approach to the treatment of Wegener's granulomatosis. *Arthritis Rheum* 1999;42:2666-73
- Reinhold-Keller E, Beuge N, Latza U, de Groot K, Rudert H, Nolle B, et al. An interdisciplinary approach to the care of patients with Wegener's granulomatosis. *Arthritis Rheum* 2000;43:1021-32

20 Laboratory tests

Margaret J Larché, David A Isenberg

This chapter describes investigations in the order they should be performed in patients with suspected rheumatological disorders. Abnormal haematological tests are found often, with anaemias and platelet abnomalities the most common. Biochemical abnormalities include raised protein and globulin levels and reflect a non-specific inflammatory response. Haematological and biochemical investigations are useful in diagnosis and monitoring, and immunological investigations are mainly used at time of diagnosis.

Haematological investigations

A full blood count and erythrocyte sedimentation rate are used to monitor disease activity, to assess the effects of drug treatment, to exclude factors such as dietary deficiency or haemolysis that may be contributing to the morbidity of a rheumatological disease, and (rarely) to exclude a primary haematological malignancy that can mimic various forms of arthritis. The erythrocyte sedimentation rate is considered in detail in the section on acute phase proteins.

Platelet abnormalities

Platelet abnormalities are seen often in rheumatic disorders, the most common is a mild to moderate thrombocytosis that correlates with disease activity. In rheumatoid arthritis, idiopathic thrombocytopenia may occur. Autoimmune thrombocytopenia (usually chronic but occasionally acute) occurs in up to 20% of patients with lupus and in patients with primary antiphospholipid antibody syndrome. In some of these patients, antiplatelet antibodies have been detected. About 15% of patients with "idiopathic" thrombocytopenia later develop lupus. Infections associated with arthralgia—for example, cytomegalovirus, hepatitis C, and HIV—can cause thrombocytopenia.

Aims of haematological investigations
- Monitor disease activity
- Assess effects of drug treatment
- Exclude factors such as dietary deficiency or haemolysis
- Exclude primary haematological malignancy

Causes of idiopathic thrombocytopenia
- Gold
- Penicillamine
- Cytotoxic drugs
    Methotrexate
    Cyclophosphamide
    Mycophenolate mofetil
- Felty's syndrome

Felty's syndrome—the association of rheumatoid arthritis with leucopenia (predominantly neutropenia) and splenomegaly (and often leg ulcers)

Anaemia and rheumatological disease

Type	Indices	Causes
Iron-deficient	• Decreased levels of serum iron • Increased total iron binding capacity • Microcytosis • Hypochromasia	• Non-steroidal anti-inflammatory drug related and corticosteroid related peptic ulcer disease • Disease—for example, oesophagitis in scleroderma

Megaloblastic	• Macrocytosis
	• Decreased levels of
	    Folate
	    Vitamin B-12
	    Thyroid function tests
		• Azathioprine
		• Methotrexate (decreased levels of folate)
		• Pernicious anaemia

Haemolytic	• Reticulocytes • Haptoglobins • Positive direct Coombs test	• Systemic lupus erythematosus • Drugs—for example, dapsone

Chronic disease	• Normochromic
	• Normocytic
	• Decreased:
	    Levels of serum levels of iron
	    Total iron binding capacity
	• Increased ferritin
		• Multifactorial
		• Decreased levels of erythropoietin
		• Abnormal erythrocyte development
		• Increased levels of cytokines—for example, interleukin-1 and tumour necrosis factor α

White blood cell abnormalities

Felty's syndrome is rare. Leucopenia, particularly lymphopenia, is common in lupus. Bone marrow suppression is a well recognised complication of immunosuppressive drugs used to treat severe rheumatoid arthritis, psoriatic arthritis, and lupus. Patients taking these drugs should have regular haematological assessments to detect bone marrow suppression early. Leucocytosis is occasionally found in flares of lupus, but is more often a reflection of prolonged neutrophil survival induced by corticosteroid treatment. Infective causes of a leucocytosis (particularly a neutrophilia) should be excluded. Less common abnormalities, such as monocytopenia and eosinophilia in rheumatoid arthritis and basopenia in lupus, are well described.

Coagulation abnormalities

Lupus anticoagulant is discussed in the section about antiphospholipid antibodies.

Acute phase response

This response is a coordinated set of systemic and local events associated with the inflammation that is the consequence of tissue damage. The term is misleading in that the changes may occur in acute and chronic inflammation. About 30 acute phase proteins are known. Raised concentrations of these proteins in serum often last for several days after the initiating event, and their synthesis in the liver is triggered by several cytokines. These cytokines derive from macrophages activated at the site of the injury, although other cell types—for example, fibroblasts and endothelial cells—are also sources. Some specificity exists in these interactions: for example, synthesis of C reactive protein depends on interleukin-6, whereas haptoglobin is influenced by all three of the cytokines described.

To measure all aspects of the acute phase response is impractical and unnecessary. The most widely used measurements are erythrocyte sedimentation rate, C reactive protein, and plasma viscosity. Less common measurements are serum amyloid A protein, haptoglobin, and fibrinogen.

Immunosuppressive drugs that can cause bone marrow suppression

- Azathioprine
- Methotrexate
- Leflunomide
- Cyclophosphamide
- Mycophenolate mofetil

Cytokines that trigger proteins of acute phase response

- Interleukin-1
- Interleukin-6
- Tumour necrosis factor α

Measurement of acute phase response

- Detects inflammatory disease
- Assesses disease activity
- Monitors therapy
- Detects intercurrent infection

Acute phase reactants

Measurement

Erythrocyte sedimentation rate

- Distance in mm that red blood cells fall in one hour
- Depends on degree of aggregation of red cells (rouleaux) and the packed cell volume
- Indirect reflection of acute phase proteins and immunoglobulins
- Plasma proteins including fibrinogen, β_2 microglobulin and immunoglobulins
- Anaemia

C reactive protein

- Immunoassay (mg/l)
- Pentameric protein released from liver under influence of interleukin-6 within four hours of tissue injury
- Large increase in infection, often normal in systemic lupus erythematosus

---

Blood test abnormalities in some rheumatological diseases

	Rheumatoid arthritis	Systemic lupus erythematosus	Polymyalgia rheumatica	Crystal arthritis	Myositis	Scleroderma	Osteoporosis	Osteomalacia
Anaemia								
• Chronic disease	++	++	+	−	−	++		
• Microcytic or hypochromic	++	+	++	−	−	++	−	−
• Megaloblastic	++	−	−	−	−	−	−	−
							−	−
Acute phase response								
• Erythrocyte sedimentation rate	++	++	+++	+/−	+	+		
• C reactive protein	+	−	+	+/−	−	−	−	−
Abnormal renal function	+	++	+/−	+	+/−	+	−	
Abnormal liver function	+	+	−	−	−		−	
Uric acid	−	−	−	+	−	−	−	
Bone biochemistry								
• Alkaline phosphatase	+	−	+	−	−	−	−	+/−
Calcium ions	−	−	−	−	−	−	−	↓/−
Phosphate ions	−	−	−	−	−	−	−	↓/−

Levels of cytokines (for example, interleukin-6, interleukin-1, and tumour necrosis factor α) in plasma may be used to assess acute phase response in the future, but now are used just as research tools. Other potentially useful tests not in general use are for serum amyloid protein A protein and matrix metalloproteinase 3—both may predict bone damage in early rheumatoid arthritis.

Biochemical investigations

Most biochemical tests are useful for monitoring organ specific complications of disease or assessing side effects of drugs.

Liver function
Abnormalities in liver function may reflect disease activity in some rheumatic diseases (for example, alkaline phosphatase activity in rheumatoid arthritis and liver transaminases in polymyositis reflecting muscle damage). Raised enzyme activities may also be due to damage from drugs used to treat rheumatic diseases. The recommended frequency of hepatic monitoring varies, but baseline assessment is advisable before starting any such drugs.

Many enzymes and proteins measured do not originate solely from the liver. Paget's disease is a common cause of an isolated rise in alkaline phosphatase activity, and in this the patient's bone is the site of origin.

Renal function
Abnormal renal function may also be a component of a rheumatic disease or a consequence of treatment. Non-steroidal anti-inflammatory drugs and methotrexate often are implicated in cases of renal dysfunction, and the dose might need to be reduced or the drug discontinued. Measurement of plasma creatinine concentration is used widely to test renal dysfunction. It is not sensitive, however: creatinine clearance must decrease to <30 ml/min (about one third of normal values) before the plasma creatinine concentration becomes abnormally high.

Plasma urea concentration is a less sensitive measure than plasma creatinine concentration and is influenced by several factors, including rate of protein metabolism and fluid balance. Patients with vasculitis in particular will often have active urinary sediment with protein or blood, or both, on dipstick testing and granular or red cell casts on microscopy of centrifuged samples.

Twenty four hour urine collections depend on the reliability of the patient, but are useful in the assessment of creatinine clearance and protein leak from the kidneys. Serial estimations of urine protein concentration help to gauge the response to treatment in, for example, patients with lupus or with amyloidosis complicating rheumatoid arthritis. An accurate measure of glomerular filtration rate, the chromium 51 labelled ethylene diamine tetraamine test is a widely available and useful assessment of glomerular function.

Bone biochemistry
The markers measured most often are serum alkaline phosphatase activity and serum levels of calcium and phosphate. All three tend to be normal in osteoporosis, but a raised alkaline phosphatase activity of bone origin is the key biochemical feature of Paget's disease. Severe cases of osteomalacia are associated with hypocalcaemia, hypophosphataemia, and increased alkaline phosphatase activity; parathyroid hormone levels may be high but vitamin D levels are usually low.

Elevated alkaline phosphatase activity

- Temporal arteritis
- Polymyalgia rheumatica
- Scleroderma
- Occasionally systemic lupus erythematosus

Drugs used to treat rheumatic disease may produce raised enzyme activity

- Methotrexate
- Azathioprine
- Cyclophosphamide
- Sulfasalazine
- Leflunomide

Assessment of urine is a simple way of monitoring renal involvement in patients with rheumatological disease

---

Main bone diseases that present to rheumatologists

- Osteoporosis
- Osteomalacia
- Paget's disease

Biological markers of bone and cartilage turnover

- Cross-linked collagen derivatives
- Pyridinoline
- Deoxypyridinoline

Biochemical markers of bone and cartilage turnover are being used in some centres as sensitive assays of bone turnover in osteoporosis. During periods of high collagen turnover, such as after the menopause, in Paget's disease, and in hyperparathyroidism, raised levels of these compounds are found in urine.

Other biochemical tests

Recent epidemiological studies suggest that patients with chronic inflammatory diseases such as rheumatoid arthritis and systemic lupus erythematosus are predisposed to atherosclerosis in a manner independent of other known risk factors. These patients should be screened for any treatable cardiovascular risk factor, such as diabetes and hyperlipidaemia. Assessment of fasting glucose and lipids should be made in all patients with chronic inflammatory diseases.

Plasma urate is discussed in Chapter 9. Muscle diseases, polymyositis particularly, are associated with a rise in activity of creatine kinase. This enzyme occurs as three isoenzymes: with the MM form originating principally in the skeletal muscle. Serial measurements of creatine kinase activity often reflect disease activity in myositis, but interpretation of readings should take into account possible racial variations and the fact that vigorous exercise and intramuscular injections can dramatically but temporarily raise enzyme activity.

Rheumatoid factors

Rheumatoid factor antibodies are immunoglobulins that bind to the Fc (constant region) of immunoglobulin G. Several tests are available, including the classic Rose-Waaler test and the latex agglutination test, which identify only the immunoglobulin M isotype. Immunoglobulin G and immunoglobulin A rheumatoid factors are detected by enzyme linked immunosorbent assay, which is becoming more widely available. Oligoarticular rheumatoid arthritis may be associated with a negative test for immunoglobulin M rheumatoid factor but a positive test for immunoglobulin G rheumatoid factor. The clinical specificity of immunoglobulin A rheumatoid factor is not clear, but it has been found early in the course of rheumatoid arthritis. Normal ranges vary between laboratories, but titres >1:80 are generally considered to be a positive result.

A raised titre of immunoglobulin M rheumatoid factor has definite but limited value as a diagnostic test for rheumatoid arthritis. The test is positive in about 70% of patients with rheumatoid arthritis and in some with other disorders, including other arthritic conditions (for example, lupus and Sjögren's syndrome), but in the right clinical context, it can be useful.

Immunological investigations

Autoantibodies

Autoantibodies are immunoglobulins that bind to self antigens (molecules present in the patient's own tissues). Low concentrations of autoantibodies are present in the plasma of normal individuals, especially in the elderly, but in autoimmune conditions some of these antibodies are overexpressed. This may result from a variety of factors, including genetic predisposition and environmental triggers, such as infection.

Raised concentrations of certain organ specific antibodies are sometimes seen in patients with rheumatic diseases (and in their relatives); this may reflect an increased tendency to autoimmunity in such individuals. Autoantibodies that are not organ specific, however, are more characteristic of these conditions. Detection of autoantibodies in patients with

---

Conditions in which rheumatoid factor is found

- Rheumatoid arthritis (70%)
- Sjögren's syndrome (about 60%)
- Systemic lupus erythematosus (25%)
- Vasculitis such as polyarteritis nodosa
- Sarcoidosis
- Infections such as infectious mononucleosis, subacute bacterial endocarditis, tuberculosis, leprosy, and syphilis (variable occurrence, up to 40% in tuberculosis)
- Malignancies such as myeloma and Waldenström's macroglobulinaemia (presenting in up to 10% of patients with myeloma)
- Cryoglobulinaemia
- Chronic liver disease
- Old age (about 5% of people aged over 69 years)

Tests for rheumatoid factor

Immunoglobulin M

Rose-Waaler test
- Relies on ability of rheumatoid factors to agglutinate sheep erythrocytes coated with antisheep immunoglobulin

Latex agglutination test
- Latex particles coated with human immunoglobulin G aggregate in presence of immunoglobulin M rheumatoid factor

Immunoglobulin G and A
- Enzyme linked immunosorbent assay

Autoantibodies may be divided into those directed against certain organ specific antigens (such as the acetylcholine receptor in myasthenia gravis and intrinsic factor in pernicious anaemia) and those that bind to more widespread antigens such as DNA or phospholipid component of cell membranes, such as cardiolipin

Autoantibodies associated with some rheumatological diseases

	Rheumatoid factor	Antinuclear antibodies	DsDNA	Ro	La	Sm	RNP	ANCA	Jo-1	Topoisomerase	Cardiolipin
• Rheumatoid arthritis	+++	+	−	+/−	+/−	−	−	−	−	−	−
• Systemic lupus erythematosus	+	+++	+++	++	++	++	++	−	−	−	++
• Sjögren's syndrome	+	++	−	+++	+++	−	−	−	−	−	−
• Myositis	−	++	−	−	−	−	−	−	+	−	−
• Systemic sclerosis	−	+	−	−		−	−	−	+	+	−
• Antiphospholipid syndrome	−	−	−	−	−	−	−	−	−	−	+++
• Vasculitides	+	−	−	−		−	−	++	−	−	−

ANCA, antineutrophil cytoplasmic antibodies; RNP, ribonuclear protein

rheumatic disorders is generally more useful for diagnosis than monitoring disease activity.

Antinuclear antibodies

These are immunoglobulins that bind to antigens in the cell nucleus. These antibodies are usually detected by immunofluorescence, using murine liver or kidney cells, or a human epithelial cell line. As with rheumatoid factor, a titre >1:80 is usually considered positive, although considerable variation exists between laboratories. A positive test for antinuclear antibodies is not diagnostic of systemic lupus erythematosus, as it may occur in several conditions, including hepatic, pulmonary, and haematological diseases, and malignancy. In infectious diseases, the test tends to be positive only transiently, but in the right clinical context, a positive test is strongly suggestive of an autoimmune rheumatic disease.

The pattern of immunofluorescence varies according to which nuclear or cytoplasmic antigens are recognised.

Antibodies to DNA

Anti-DNA antibodies are detected by several methods including the radioimmunoassay or Farr test, enzyme linked immunosorbent assay, and immunofluorescence test with the haemoflagellated organism, *Crithidia luciliae*.

Crithidia contains pure double stranded DNA in a very large mitochondrion, so a positive assay is virtually specific to patients with lupus. Double stranded DNA antibodies are often found in high levels in lupus and are especially likely to be found in patients with renal disease. They may reflect disease activity, and a rise in titre can predict a flare. The development of positive double stranded DNA autoantibodies after treatment with the anti-tumour necrosis factor α monoclonal antibody, infliximab, in patients with rheumatoid arthritis has been recorded. These antibodies are predominantly of the immunoglobulin M subtype and are associated rarely with a lupus-like syndrome. Other drug induced lupus syndromes are characterised by the presence of anti-histone antibodies.

Antibodies to extractable nuclear antigens

These antibodies, such as Ro, La, Sm, ribonuclear protein, centromere, and topoisomerase, can be detected by counterimmunoelectrophoresis, in which serum is tested against a saline extract of mammalian nuclei and compared with reference sera to determine a line of precipitation. More specific tests for each antigen (which consist of varying combinations of RNA and protein) are now available in many laboratories and are generally based on immunoblot or enzyme

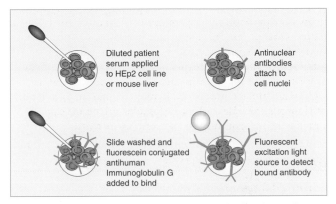

Indirect immunofluorescence for antinuclear antibodies. Serum from patients is diluted in serial doubling dilutions. A titre of 1:80 means that the patient's serum has been diluted by a factor of 80. The human epithelial 2 cell line is derived from human epithelial cells that are cultured as a monolayer

Patterns of antinuclear antibody staining: associations with immunological disease

Pattern	Antigen	Disease associations
Homogeneous	DNA or histone proteins	Systemic lupus erythematosus
Speckled	RNA and Sm, Ro, and La proteins	Sjögren's syndrome, overlap syndromes
Nucleolar	Nucleolar proteins	Scleroderma
Centromeric	Proteins in centromere	Cutaneous scleroderma

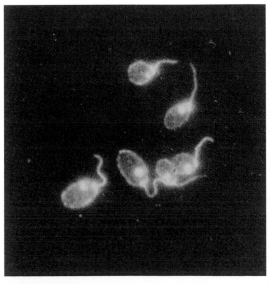

Crithidia staining

107

linked immunosorbent assays. The identification of antibodies to one or more antigen in a patient's serum can be helpful in the diagnosis of an autoimmune disease.

Antifilaggrin antibodies

Antibodies to proteins involved in epithelial cell differentiation, known as filaggrins are found in patients with rheumatoid arthritis. More recently, antibodies to citrullinated peptides that react with anti-filaggrin antibodies have been found to be 95% specific for rheumatoid arthritis. Enzyme linked immunosorbent assays often are used for research purposes to detect such antibodies, but they are not measured routinely in most immunology laboratories.

Antiphospholipid antibodies

In the rheumatological context, antiphospholipid antibodies bind chiefly to negatively charged phospholipids such as cardiolipin. Four tests are available.

Persistently raised concentrations of antiphospholipid antibodies (notably of the immunoglobulin G isotype) are associated with several clinical features, including thrombosis (both arterial and venous), recurrent fetal loss, thrombocytopenia, and various neurological disorders. Antiphospholipid syndrome may occur in isolation or in the context of a connective tissue disease such as lupus. Some evidence shows that these antibodies may directly interfere with coagulation mechanisms.

Antineutrophil cytoplasmic antibodies

These are antibodies that bind to antigens in the cytoplasm of neutrophils; they are found often in patients with vasculitides. The standard test is immunofluorescence on cultured neutrophils.

Cytoplasmic antineutrophil cytoplasmic antibodies and peripheral antineutrophil cytoplasmic antibodies bind to several proteins, the most common being serine proteinase 3 and myeloperoxidase. Solid phase immunoassays may be used to determine the specificity in each case.

Antibodies to serine proteinase 3 are found in about 80% of patients with Wegener's granulomatosis. Antibodies against myeloperoxidase are common in polyarteritis nodosa but have also been identified in patients with vasculitis as a complication of lupus, rheumatoid arthritis, and bowel diseases such as ulcerative colitis. Antibodies with other specificities have been described in non-vasculitic diseases—for example, inflammatory bowel disease and autoimmune hepatitis—but they are of limited value.

Immunoglobulins

A general polyclonal rise in total immunoglobulin concentrations is often seen in many inflammatory rheumatic diseases as a non-specific reflection of an acute phase response. In Sjögren's syndrome, total immunoglobulin concentrations may be substantially raised—often up to 30 g/l or more. Regular estimates of immunoglobulins and determination of their subtype by protein electrophoresis should be performed in these patients, as they have an approximately 40 times increased risk of lymphoma.

Complement

Proteins of the complement cascade play a central role in cell lysis, opsonisation of bacteria, and clearance of immune complexes. The C3 and C4 components are measured most often (and in some laboratories CH50, which is a measure of total activity of the whole complement pathway) and are useful when screening for complement deficiencies.

Four tests available for antiphospholipid antibodies

- The lupus anticoagulant test is the most sensitive test in current use. It measures the ability of antiphospholipid antibodies to prolong clotting and is based on the partial thromboplastin time
- The simplest and cheapest is the enzyme linked immunosorbent assay for anticardiolipin antibodies. This allows detection and quantitation of immunoglobulin G and immunoglobulin M antibodies against cardiolipin
- The Venereal Disease Research Laboratory test, which is used to test for syphilis, uses a variety of phospholipids. Antibodies in test plasma may bind to these and create a false positive test for syphilis. This test is of limited diagnostic value
- A fourth overlapping population of antiphospholipid antibodies comprises antibodies to a cofactor binding protein, such as β_2 glycoprotein I. Assays for immunoglobulin anti-β_2 glycoprotein I, which may have utility as an adjunctive marker of future thrombotic or neurological events in patients with systemic lupus erythematosus and antiphospholipid syndrome, are becoming available at specialist centres

---

Patterns seen in standard immunofluorescence test for antineutrophil cytoplasmic antibodies

- Diffuse "cytoplasmic" staining
- "Peripheral or perinuclear" staining pattern around the edge of the nucleus

---

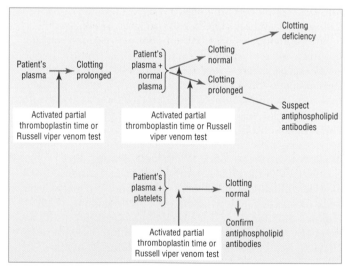

Detection of lupus anticoagulant. Although lupus anticoagulant is associated with thrombotic episodes in vivo, paradoxically the in vitro test relies on prolongation of activated partial thromboplastin time (or Russell viper venom test, or the Kaolin Cephalin clotting time). This is thought to be because of the interaction with the phospholipid portion of the prothrombin activator complex of the clotting cascade. When patient's plasma is added to normal plasma, the clotting factors are replenished and, if the prolongation of clotting is caused by a deficiency of a clotting factor, this will be corrected: however, if antiphospholipid antibodies are the cause of the abnormal test result, this will not be corrected. An excess of phospholipids is then added in the form of platelets, and this should correct the clotting prolongation

Complement degradation products—particularly C3d and C4d—are being used as research tools as markers of disease activity of systemic lupus erythematosus.

Genetic associations

Genetic factors play a role in many of the rheumatological diseases. Most are polygenic in nature, however, and analysis of genetic markers is of limited value. Close associations between human leucocyte antigens are found with diseases such as ankylosing spondylitis and rheumatoid arthritis. In the former, 95% of patients possess a human leucocyte antigen-B27 allele. The frequency of B27 in the general population is around 10%. Human leucocyte antigen typing is expensive, however, and it is unnecessary in most instances for several reasons:

- thorough clinical assessment with relevant haematological, biochemical, immunological, and radiological investigations will enable a clear diagnosis to be made
- human leucocyte antigen haplotypes are not associated specifically with individual rheumatological diseases
- in families with existing ankylosing spondylitis the positive predictive value of B27 is reduced.

Microbiology

The differential diagnosis in any acute monoarthropathy must include septic arthritis, which is excluded easily by joint aspiration and culture of synovial fluid and blood. The laboratory should be told if tuberculosis or gonococcus are suspected, as specific culture media and techniques are needed. Polyarthropathies may be associated with several viral and bacterial infections. Chronic infection with hepatitis B or C may cause polyarthralgia. Acute rheumatic fever (which is still a major killer on a worldwide scale, but is rare in the western world) is associated with a positive test for antistreptolysin-O and *Streptococcus* species in blood and throat cultures. The seronegative spondyloarthropathies often are related temporally to diarrhoeal illnesses or urethritis. Parvovirus B19 has been associated with a self-limiting polyarthritis similar to rheumatoid arthritis. Other viruses such as rubella, human T-lymphotropic virus, and HIV may present with arthralgia. Lyme disease is associated with a rash and polyarthropathy, and the diagnosis depends on finding antibodies to the spirochaete *Borrelia burgdorferi* in serum.

Conclusion

Blood tests are useful for assessment, diagnosis, and monitoring of rheumatological diseases. The trend is for laboratories (particularly in the United States) to use "rheumatology screens" with an array of markers often including rheumatoid factor, antinuclear antibody, erythrocyte sedimentation rate, and C reactive protein. This is not to be recommended as it leads to many false positive results. Blood tests should be used judiciously where indicated.

Changes in complement in different rheumatological diseases

Change in C3, C4, or CH50	Characteristic conditions	Cause
Large increase	Bacterial infections	Part of acute phase response
Increase	Inflammatory diseases including rheumatoid arthritis and seronegative arthritides	Part of acute phase response
Decrease	Systemic lupus erythematosus, especially lupus nephritis, other vasculitides	Consumption by immune complexes
Decrease	Hereditary hypocomplementaemic syndromes	Hereditary

Organisms implicated in diarrhoeal diseases and urethritis

- Salmonella
- Yersinia
- Campylobacter
- Chlamydia

Further reading

- Shipley M, Black CM, Compston J, O'Grabaigh D. Rheumatology. In: Kumar P, Clark M. *Clinical medicine.* 5th ed. Philadelphia: WB Saunders, 2002
- Hakim G, Clunie A. *Oxford handbook of rheumatology.* Oxford: Oxford University Press, 2002
- Playfair JHL, Lydyard PM. *Medical immunology made memorable.* Edinburgh: Churchill Livingstone, 2000
- Klippel JH, Dieppe PA. *Rheumatology.* St Louis: Mosby International, 1997

21   The team approach

Janet Cushnaghan, Jackie McDowell

The patient's journey

The terms "musculoskeletal disorders" and "rheumatological disorders" are used to describe diseases that affect the joints, bones, soft tissue, and muscles. Many types of rheumatological diseases exist, and many types of clinicians will be involved in the care of affected individuals. Some conditions also affect other organs and systems, which makes complex management necessary. The severity of musculoskeletal conditions ranges from mild and self-limiting to life-threatening. The management of many patients can be undertaken in the primary care setting, but others benefit from the expertise and management of a specialist hospital unit. In this chapter, we will look at the personnel who contribute to the management of a patient with inflammatory arthritis throughout the healthcare system.

The importance of a whole team or multidisciplinary team approach between primary and secondary care with the patient at the core cannot be overemphasised. Every aspect of treatment is as important as the next, and the combination of all elements leads to successful management.

At different stages of each condition, different members of the team will provide individual specialist skills. An understanding, by all those involved, of the individual roles of all members is vital. To know who can provide what and when comes with experience. One clinician should take a lead role or have an overview of the management plan for individual patients. This may not always be the consultant—it may be a therapist or nurse. Communication between all members of the team must be open and easy.

A "joined up service" that provides seamless care between primary and secondary care is possible with good communication, cascading of information, and clear evidence based guidelines or care pathways for management. Focus and effort allow the creation of high quality, evidence based, cost effective plans for individualised patient care that use time productively. For such guidelines or care pathways to be effective, all individuals involved must have ownership, be involved in team collaboration, and participate actively in their development. Guidelines to facilitate best practice in the United Kingdom guidelines have been developed.

The Scottish Intercollegiate Guidelines Network (www.sign.ac.uk) (check, and add date accessed) produced an outstanding example of what can be achieved with quality collaborative multidisciplinary teamwork with their Management of Early Rheumatoid Arthritis National Clinical Guideline for Scotland.[1]

The Arthritis and Musculoskeletal Alliance (formerly known as British League Against Rheumatism) is an umbrella organisation that brings together a variety of national societies concerned with rheumatic and musculoskeletal diseases. In 1997, British League Against Rheumatism developed standards of care for patients with osteoarthritis and rheumatoid arthritis that they believe provide the optimum level of service that a person with osteoarthritis and rheumatoid arthritis should

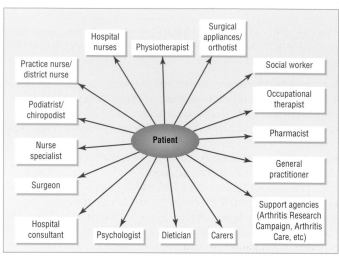

Diagram showing the diversity of personnel involved in the team

---

Guidelines or care pathways

Guidelines or care pathways should be:
- distributed widely
- available freely to all relevant personnel
- easily accessible in appropriate or varied formats
    hard copies
    internet
    intranet

Scottish Intercollegiate Guidelines Network

Inform standards for practice for:
- Rheumatologists
- General practitioners
- Rheumatology nurse specialists
- Physiotherapists
- Occupational therapists
- Dieticians
- Podiatrists
- Pharmacists
Aims to:
- Ensure guidelines adopted after local discussion
- Ensure guidelines used for derivation of specific local guidelines to implement the national guidelines in individual hospitals, units, and practices
- Secure compliance with national guidelines

receive. The standards cover primary care, rheumatology secondary care, and orthopaedic secondary care, but standards for some community care issues, as well as issues across society, such as physical access, are also included. British League Against Rheumatism divided the standards into two categories:

- essential standards
- desirable standards.

Members of the management team

Below we consider the roles of some, but not all, members of the team and how they may be involved in the care of patients with rheumatological disease.

General practitioners

The general practitioner is in most cases the "gatekeeper" for the patient, and general practitioners' knowledge and experience of rheumatology are variable. A consistent approach is vital in the management of rheumatology patients, however, no matter where in the country they live or to whom they present. Where good communication links have been developed between primary and secondary care and guidelines exist, the general practitioner will be confident in identifying patients who need to be referred to the specialist unit. The general practitioner will also be familiar with what information and prior investigation or treatment is permissible, and what information is helpful or not helpful for the rheumatologist for the patient's initial consultation.

After the onset of symptoms, a patient presents to his or her general practitioner for examination and any necessary investigations. A careful history and physical examination are the most important components of a rheumatological assessment. Local clinical guidelines, where available, will inform the referral pattern.

Consultant rheumatologists

After referral by a general practitioner or other colleague, a rheumatologist will see a patient, make a diagnosis, and initiate a management plan. After this, some people can be managed in the community with occasional extra advice from the rheumatologist, but others will need ongoing follow up by the hospital department due to the complexity of their condition or its treatment. Most people will enter into a shared care arrangement, however, in which the hospital provides guidelines as to the monitoring of the condition and its treatment to be carried out in the community and the person will be reviewed occasionally by the hospital department. The British Society for Rheumatology has produced guidelines on the monitoring of second line drugs for inflammatory arthritis, which can be adapted to local needs but form the starting point for individual agreements between primary and secondary care.

Physiotherapists

The physiotherapist aims to relieve pain, maintain movement and muscle strength, and thereby maintain function and quality of life. Several techniques are available to fulfil these aims. The physiotherapist, along with most other members of the team, aims to equip the patient with the relevant knowledge of their condition, the appropriate skills needed to manage it, and the right attitude to come to terms with and cope with the condition. The patient is given an active role in their own management and gains a feeling of control over their condition. This self-management approach has been shown to reduce pain and reduce the demands made on the healthcare system, such as fewer visits to medical practitioners.

Essential standards in primary care for osteoarthritis and rheumatoid arthritis

The general practitioner should:
- Discuss the nature of arthritis at an early stage—applies to OA and RA
- Examine the joints at an early stage—applies to OA and RA
- Explain the role of the following as possible treatments
  Exercise—applies to OA and RA
  Weight control—applies to OA and RA
  Footwear or chiropody—applies to OA
  Painkilling medication—applies to OA and RA
  Anti-inflammatory (first-line/non-steroidal anti-inflammatory) drugs—applies to OA and RA
  Antirheumatic (second-line/disease modifying antirheumatic) drugs—applies to RA
  Oral steroids—applies to RA
  Steroid injection—applies to RA
  Physiotherapy—applies to RA
- Explain the role of the following in helping with treatment
  Hospital (rheumatology or orthopaedic department) in the treatment and care of arthritis—applies to RA

OA=osteoarthritis; RA=rheumatoid arthritis

Check list of desirable standards for in primary care for osteoarthritis and rheumatoid arthritis

The general practitioner should:
- Explain the role of the following as possible treatments
  Physiotherapy—applies to OA
  Steroid injection—applies to OA
  Footwear and chiropody—applies to RA
- Explain the role of the following in helping with treatment
  Hospital (rheumatology or orthopaedic department)—applies to OA
  Social worker—applies to OA and RA
  Someone able to discuss personal or sexual relationships—applies to OA and RA
  Rheumatology nurse practitioner—applies to RA
- Provide written information on the following
  Arthritis in general—applies to OA and RA
  Medication being taken for arthritis—applies to OA and RA
  Exercise—applies to OA and RA
  Voluntary self-help and support groups—applies to OA and RA
  Self-management courses—applies to OA and RA

OA=osteoarthritis; RA=rheumatoid arthritis

United Kingdom Primary Care Rheumatology Society has an interest in the specialty in general practice and the community and offers a distance learning package www.pcrsociety.com Telephone: 01609 774794

Aims of physiotherapy
- To relieve pain
- To maintain movement and muscle strength
- To maintain function and quality of life

Physiotherapy techniques

Electrotherapy
- Used to reduce pain, which in turn allows more movement and hence improved function

Hot and cold therapies, including hydrotherapy
- May be beneficial for:
  Increasing muscle strength
  Improving joint motion
  Improving gait

Occupational therapists

Throughout the course of a disease, the occupational therapist strives to maintain functional independence of the individual by whatever means. Many occupational therapists work in the community and can assist with adaptations to the environment and applications for grants to help finance this.

Nurse specialists

Many rheumatology departments now include a nurse specialist who fulfils many roles, including education and counselling, monitoring the toxicity of various treatments, and monitoring and managing disease over time. This role has a large liaison aspect to it and will bridge the gap between primary and secondary care. The relationship that builds between practitioner and patient is very important and can help patients cope, as many of the conditions are chronic. In some departments this "specialist" role may be undertaken by other allied health professionals such as a physiotherapist or an occupational therapist. Many of these extended role practitioners undertake tasks such as intra-articular injections or alteration of doses of drugs as part of the management plan for these patients. Allied health professionals are constantly extending their roles; drug prescribing, for example, will soon be a routine aspect of this work. Research has shown the nurse practitioner to be as effective as a medical doctor in the care of patients with inflammatory arthritis.

Podiatrist, chiropodist, or orthotist

Podiatrists are increasingly becoming recognised as important members of the team. Many rheumatological conditions affect the feet and make walking painful. The podiatrist's role is to prevent deformity, maintain comfort and function of the feet, and provide education and advice about foot care and appropriate footwear.

Education groups

Education programmes can reduce pain and disability and even reduce the number of visits to specialists. If the patient is given the knowledge to cope with their condition and carry out self-management they can be put in control of their disease. People equipped with coping strategies can make their own choices as to how their disease is managed. Programmes led by trained lay people are as effective as those run by professionals. Arthritis is not "special," and strategies for coping are the same as those needed for any chronic disease. Many groups now include people with respiratory conditions or cardiovascular conditions, and the same approach of goal setting and problem solving works for all.

Support agencies

Many support agencies exist for arthritis and associated conditions. These fulfil varying roles—from fund raising to the welfare of people with the conditions. People may benefit from literature provided by these groups, support given to them and their families, provision of adapted hotels, and the benefits of the scientific research that they have funded.

It has not been possible to focus on every single professional that may be involved in the complex care of patients with a rheumatological condition. We hope we have highlighted the philosophy of care that can be adapted to suit all conditions and embrace all members of the multidisciplinary team. A wide diversity of input is needed, and this needs the involvement of a diversity of people.

Occupational therapists

Provide
- Splints (resting or working)
- "Gadgets" to help with activities of daily living
- Adaptations to the home or work environment

Educate with advice on:
- Joint protection
- Pacing
- Relaxation

Role of nurse specialist

- Education and counselling
- Monitoring the toxicity of various treatments
- Monitoring and managing disease over time
- Telephone helpline to provide advice and information for:
     Patients and carers
     Community staff
     Other members of management team
- Patient advocate
- Support for patient, family, and carers over many years
- Drug prescribing in future

A to Z of rheumatology: the team approach

A—Advice (evidence based), assessment (consistent), administration (medication), AIDS, advanced practice, audit (of practice), access (to services) appliance (fitter), Arthritis Research Campaign, arthritis care

B—Body image, biomechanics, benefits, British Society for Rheumatology, British Health Professionals in Rheumatology

C—Counselling, consistency, chronicity, carers, compliance, coping strategies, community team, clinics and combined clinics, coordination of care and services, communication, conferences, consultant (doctors and nurses)

D—Diagnosis, discharge planning, drugs, disability, diet, development (professional)

E—Equipment, empowerment, expectations, exercise, education, examination (consistent), evidence based practice

F—Flare, fatigue, follow up

G—Groups (patient and professional), general practitioner, guidelines

H—Holistic, helplines, health visitor (do more than just children)

I—Information, investigation, interventions (medical and non-medical), internet

J—Joint protection, journals (patient and professional)

K—Knowledge

L—Literature (patient), liaison.

M—Multidisciplinary, mobility, management (disease or patient), medication, monitoring (disease or patient)

N—Networking, new treatments, nurse led

O—Outcome, occupational therapy, orthotics, outpatients

P—Primary care, professional development, professional organisations, pain management, pacing, philosophy of care, podiatry, psychological and psychologist, physiotherapy, pharmacist, primary care rheumatology

Q—Questionnaires

R—Research (evidence base), retraining officers, responsibility, rest, roles (primary care team, orthotist, psychologist, physiotherapist, occupational therapy, medical staff, rheumatologist, specialist nurse, dietician, pharmacist, etc)

S—Surgery, support, social implications, self-management, secondary care, shared care, sexuality, seamless care, support groups, social workers

T—Teamwork, tertiary care, teaching, treatments

U—Unity

V—Vocation advisors, voluntary organisations

W—Work (employment)

1 Scottish Intercollegiate Guidelines Network. *Management of Early Arthritis—A National Clinical Guideline. Publication No. 48.* Edinburgh: SIGN Executive, Royal College of Physicians, 2000

Further reading

- British League Against Rheumatism. *Disability and arthritis, report of a survey.* London: British League Against Rheumatism, 1994
- British League Against Rheumatism. *Arthritis—getting it right. A guide for planners.* London: British League against Rheumatism, 1997
- British Society of Rheumatology. *Musculoskeletal disorders: providing for the patient's needs. A basis for planning a rheumatology service.* London: British Society of Rheumatology, 1994
- British Society of Rheumatology. *BSR guidelines for second line drug monitoring.* London: British Society of Rheumatology, 2000
- Hill J, Ryan S. *A handbook for community nurses.* London: Whurr Publishers Ltd, 2000
- Le-Gallez P. *Rheumatology for nurses: patient care.* London: Whurr Publishers Ltd, 1998

22 Epidemiology of rheumatic diseases

Alex J MacGregor, Timothy D Spector

Musculoskeletal diseases account for one third of the physical disability that is experienced in the community in the United Kingdom and have an economic cost that exceeds that of heart disease and cancer. The most common single cause of disability is osteoarthritis, which can affect the knee, spine, and hip. Osteoporosis that leads to fracture is the second greatest public health problem: more than one in three women are likely to have an osteoporotic fracture at the wrist, hip, or spine during their lifetime. Rheumatoid arthritis accounts for up to 50% of the workload of rheumatologists in the United Kingdom. Although the likelihood of disability is greater with rheumatoid arthritis than osteoarthritis, seven times more people are disabled because of osteoarthritis. The connective tissue diseases, although much rarer, are often associated with considerable mortality, particularly in the young.

Rheumatoid arthritis

This disease affects women three times more often than men. Its prevalence is reported as 0.5-1% in many diverse populations worldwide. Notable exceptions exist, however: a high prevalence has been recorded in certain Native American groups, and the disease seems to be absent in rural Africa. In both men and women, the incidence increases with advancing age, although it seems to decline in very elderly people. A number of studies have reported a declining incidence of disease over the last 30 years, although recent reports suggest this fall has not been dramatic. Twin studies confirm a substantial genetic contribution: rheumatoid arthritis has a heritability of 50-60%—part of which is explained by genes that encode human leucocyte antigen-DRB1 molecules. First degree relatives of affected people are at a threefold increased risk of developing the disease themselves. This risk is approximately sixfold higher in those possessing "at risk" human leucocyte antigen-DRB1 genotypes.

Environmental factors also are likely to be important, but few strong reported associations have been replicated. Those that have been commonly implicated include a protective effect of the contraceptive pill, parity as opposed to nulliparity, and breastfeeding. Immunological evidence that points to an infectious trigger is not supported by epidemiological data. No clear clustering has been found in incident cases, and no links have been found with previous childhood diseases, size of households, or number of siblings. Immunisation has been linked with rheumatoid arthritis in case reports, but the association is unconfirmed. Altered immune responsiveness may account for the recent observation of an association between prior blood transfusion and development of disease. A negative association with schizophrenia has been reported.

Many studies report twofold to threefold increased mortality in patients with rheumatoid arthritis. In one hospital series, patients with rheumatoid arthritis had a worse survival rate at five years than age matched cases with Hodgkin's disease or triple vessel cardiovascular disease. In terms of morbidity, patients are suggested to be less severely affected by their disease than they were 30-50 years ago. Current estimates are

Ranking of top three reasons for general practice consultations

	45-64	Age (years) 65-74	≥75
Men	Respiratory	Circulatory	Circulatory
	Musculoskeletal	Respiratory	Respiratory
	Circulatory	Musculoskeletal	Musculoskeletal
Women	Musculoskeletal	Circulatory	Circulatory
	Respiratory	Musculoskeletal	Musculoskeletal
	Mental	Respiratory	Respiratory

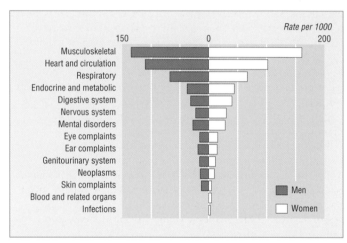

Prevalence of chronic sickness in the United Kingdom

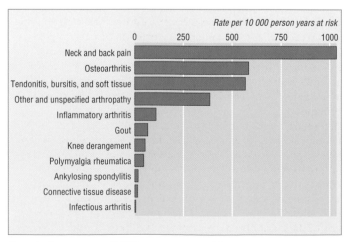

Consultation rates per 10 000 person years at risk

114

that about one third of patients who attend a specialist clinic will be moderately or severely disabled in ten years, one third will be slightly disabled, and one third will maintain normal function. Patients are at higher risk of developing myeloma and lymphomas, but this does not seem to be related to their underlying treatment.

Osteoarthritis

Osteoarthritis is one of the most common of all diseases and is extremely dependent on age. Below the age of 40 years, <5% of people have any evidence of disease; by the age of 75, >70% will have radiological features of the disease. The disease has a worldwide occurrence, although the sites most often affected vary in different populations. Osteoarthritis of the knee is the most common cause of disability and affects locomotor function in 10% of the population aged over 50 years. The disease often first manifests between 45 and 55 years in women, in whom it is three times more common than in men.

Obesity is the major risk factor for osteoarthritis of the knee, particularly in middle aged women, in whom every 5 kg increase in weight increases their risk by 30%. Other known risk factors include extensive knee bending and previous knee injuries such as meniscectomy. Long periods of participation in weight-bearing sports also increase the risk.

Osteoarthritis of the hip is less common than that of the knee, but it is more likely to cause disability. The prevalence of the disease is less than 3% in people aged up to 65 years and increases to 5% in people in their 80s. Obesity is only a minor risk factor for the disease at the hip. Strong occupational associations exist, however—for example, a fivefold increased risk above that of the general population is reported in farmers who perform long-term carrying and lifting. Acetabular dysplasia is unlikely to be responsible for more than a small percentage of cases.

A strong genetic influence on osteoarthritis at the hand, knee, and the hip has recently been established by twin and family studies, with heritabilities in the range 50-60%. Although bone density is increased in osteoarthritis, the risk of fracture is increased, which suggests that the new bone formed in osteoarthritis is abnormal. Low vitamin D levels have been implicated in the disease.

Osteoporosis

The main consequence of osteoporosis is fracture. Colles' fracture affects 15% of women and vertebral fractures up to 20% (most are asymptomatic). The most serious, however, is hip fracture, which affects one in four women who live to the age of 85 years; the lifetime risk is 15%. A quarter of these elderly patients die within a year, and more than half remain permanently disabled. The principal risk factors for hip fracture are those that contribute to (a) lack of bone strength or frailty, such as early menopause, family history, smoking, low body weight, female sex, chronic diseases, high bone turnover, and use of corticosteroids, and (b) an increase in the risk of falling, such as increased age, postural instability, dementia, lack of muscle strength, visual impairment, and concomitant medication. For each standard deviation reduction in bone density, the risk of fracture increases two to threefold. Genetic factors have an important influence on a range of factors related to fracture risk. Bone density itself has a heritability of up to 80%. Other predictive factors independent of bone density are bone turnover, bone architecture (measured by ultrasound), and the length of the femoral neck. A personal

---

Rheumatoid arthritis: risk and protection factors
- Female sex
- Positive family history
- Presence of human leucocyte antigens-DR4 and DR1
- Nulliparity
- Breastfeeding
- Use of contraceptive pill (negative association)
- Blood transfusion (positive association)
- Schizophrenia (negative association)

Risk factors for osteoarthritis

Knee
- Female sex
- Obesity
- Family history
- Knee injury
- Knee surgery
- Hand osteoarthritis
- Hormone replacement therapy (negative association)

Hip
- Male sex
- Physical activity
- Farming
- Family history

The natural course of osteoarthritis is variable. By the time patients attend a clinic, only about one third will continue to progress radiologically over the next ten years. Factors that affect progression are unclear, but they include obesity, Heberden's nodes, disease in the contralateral joint, malalignment at the knee, and evidence of subclinical inflammation

---

Risk factors for hip fracture
- Low bone density
- Family history
- Elderly females
- Thin build
- Previous fractures
- Smoking
- Early menopause
- Inactivity
- Chronic inflammation
- Corticosteroids
- Risk of falling

and family history of fracture predict the future risk of fracture. Preventive measures include increasing the amount of exercise, reducing cigarette smoking, and taking calcium and vitamin D supplements in elderly people. The long-term role of hormone replacement therapy in prevention is less clear than previously thought, as bisphosphonates are now the drug of choice in preventing new fractures.

Ankylosing spondylitis

The prevalence of ankylosing spondylitis in white European people is about 1.5 per 1000. Worldwide variations in prevalence are marked: the frequency in black Americans is one quarter that in white people. The disease is rare in Africa and Japan, but it is frequent in Native American indigenous groups. More than 90% of patients with the disease have human leucocyte antigen-B27, and the variation in disease occurrence is reflected partly by differences in the prevalence of this marker between population groups. Human leucocyte antigen-B27 on its own is not enough to cause the disease, so an infectious agent such as *Klebsiella, Shigella,* or *Yersinia* is likely to act as a trigger. Genes other than human leucocyte antigen-B27 may be involved in determination of the severity of the disease.

Ankylosing spondylitis occurs three times more commonly in males than females, but if only mild disease is considered the prevalence is equal, as males are prone to more severe disease. The mean time from onset of symptoms to radiographic diagnosis is about eight years. The disease has considerable morbidity, although more than 20% of patients can continue working normally after 20 years of disease. No marked increase in mortality is seen.

Reiter's syndrome and reactive arthritis

Reiter's syndrome is considered here to include the occurrence of synovitis after gastrointestinal and genitourinary infection. It has an estimated prevalence of less than one in 10 000 and an annual incidence of 3-30 per 100 000. The incidence is higher in the fourth decade and in men, with a men:women ratio of 3-5 : 1. The risk of disease varies according to the trigger; it is estimated at around 1% for non-gonococcal urethritis and *Salmonella, Shigella* and *Campylobacter* infections, but it has been as high as 30% in some outbreaks of *Yersinia* infection. Human leucocyte antigen-B27 confers a 50-fold risk of disease and is present in 65-96% of cases. The association with human leucocyte antigen-B27 and a high rate of epidemic infections accounts for the syndrome's increased frequency in some ethnic groups, including certain native Indians. Reiter's syndrome is also more common in homosexual men and bisexuals, in whom the increased incidence has been attributed to a higher frequency of genitourinary and gastrointestinal infections. Long term sequelae (most often recurrent arthritis, persistent foot deformities, and the development of ankylosing spondylitis) may occur in as many as 50% of patients. Human leucocyte antigen-B27 is a risk factor for severe and progressive disease.

Psoriatic arthritis

Psoriatic arthritis has a prevalence of about 0.1%, with an equal sex distribution. Epidemiologists continue to debate whether the disease is a distinct entity or is the chance occurrence of psoriasis (which itself affects 3% of the population) and

Prevalence of ankylosing spondylitis and human leucocyte antigen-B27

Ankylosing spondylitis	Prevalence (per 1000)	Human leucocyte antigen-B27	Prevalence (%)
European whites	1.5	United Kingdom	8
American Haida Indians	60	American Indian	50
Nigeria	0.8	West Africa	3

Ankylosing spondylitis occurs three times more often in men than women, but if only mild disease is considered the prevalence is equal, as males are prone to more severe disease

Epidemiology of Reiter's syndrome

- Prevalence: one per 10 000
- Incidence: 3-30 per 10 000
- Human leucocyte antigen-B27 antigen:
   Confers 50-fold risk
   Found in three quarters of patients with Reiter's syndrome
   Associated with severe and progressive disease

Epidemiology of psoriatic arthritis

Condition	Prevalence (%)
Psoriasis prevalence	3
Psoriatic arthritis prevalence	0.1
Arthritis predates psoriasis	10
Simultaneous onset	10

Epidemiologists continue to debate whether psoriatic arthritis is a distinct entity or the chance occurrence of psoriasis and inflammatory rheumatic disease inflammatory rheumatic disease. Support for considering it as a separate disease comes from longitudinal studies of patients with psoriasis. Patients who develop inflammatory arthritis are more likely to be seronegative for rheumatoid factor and have involvement of the distal interphalangeal joints—both of these are recognised clinically as distinguishing features of psoriatic arthritis. Patients with psoriasis also seem to be at increased risk of developing arthritis. A familial predisposition to the disease exists, with an approximate 40-fold increased risk in first degree relatives of affected people. Offspring with an affected father are at increased risk when compared with those with an affected mother. Associations have been reported with the human leucocyte antigens B13, B17, and Cw6, which are associated with psoriasis. An association exists with human leucocyte antigen-B27, which reflects the occurrence of spondylitic arthropathy. Among potential environmental triggers, an infectious cause is suggested by the observation that the disease develops after HIV infection. Prior trauma has also been associated with the development of the disease.

> A familial predisposition to psoriatic arthritis exists, with an approximate 40-fold increased risk in first degree relatives of affected people. Offspring with an affected father are at increased risk when compared with those with an affected mother

Gout

The prevalence of gout varies markedly between different populations. Current estimates in men are between 1 and 2%. Gout is far more common in men than women in all populations. Rural populations tend to have lower rates than those in towns. The highest rates of gout in the world are in Polynesian Islanders—for example, 10% in male Micronesians from Nauru. Black African groups have a complete absence of gout in most studies. Migrants to western societies have higher rates than in their native populations, which suggests that a combination of dietary, lifestyle, and genetic factors is involved.

Some evidence shows that the incidence of gout has increased in Europe and the United States over the last 30-40 years, which parallels an increase in serum uric acid concentrations. The major risk factor for gout is hyperuricaemia. Men generally have higher levels of uric acid than women. Alcohol intake is associated with uric acid levels, although the relation with clinical gout is not clearcut in a number of studies. Specific associations have been found with the consumption of "moonshine" whisky, which is distilled in car radiators, and wine stored in lead crystal containers.

Gout itself is not fatal but its association with obesity, hypertension, and coronary artery disease is often associated indirectly with early death.

Prevalence of gout

Men	Prevalence (%)
European	1-2
Micronesian	10
Jamaican	0.8
Black African	<0.1
Women	
All	0.2-0.5

Risk factors for gout

- Hyperuricaemia
- Obesity
- Hypertension
- Occupational exposure to lead
- Alcohol

Polymyalgia rheumatica

From an epidemiological perspective, polymyalgia rheumatica and giant cell arteritis seem to represent a single entity: 30% of cases have features of both disorders. The exact frequency of these conditions is difficult to ascertain. Estimates of prevalence in the over 50s vary between 0.2 and 10 per 1000.

Evidence shows a geographical variation. A low incidence is reported in Israel and the south of the United States; the highest recorded incidence is in southern Norway. Evidence also shows clustering within families, but large studies are sparse. No strong or consistent reports show an association with specific genetic markers. A contribution from environmental factors is suggested by evidence of seasonal clustering, with most but not all studies showing a peak in the summer. A ten-year cyclical pattern in incidence also has been reported. No infectious trigger has been identified. No clear increase in mortality is attributable to the disease, although the risk of blindness is high even in those who have taken corticosteroids.

> Polymyalgia rheumatica is exceptionally rare in people under the age of 50 years. The incidence increases dramatically between the sixth and seventh decades and declines in people aged over 80 years. The condition is more common in women at all ages

Systemic lupus erythematosus

The prevalence of systemic lupus erythematosus is about 0.03%. The frequency is high in African Americans and Afro-Caribbeans, who are at a threefold to fourfold increased risk. The prevalence of the disease in West African countries, however, is low. In most populations, the disease is nine times more common in women than men. The most common age of onset is 35-45 years. All studies have shown increased mortality, and rates are highest in ethnic minorities and poor socioeconomic groups.

A strong genetic contribution is seen: an eightfold increase in risk is reported in those who have a first degree relative with the disease, and higher concordance rates are seen in identical twins than non-identical twins. Associations have been reported with several alleles for human leucocyte antigens, although considerable heterogeneity exists between populations. Recent linkage analyses have implicated chromosomal regions outside the human leucocyte antigen, with particular interest focused on chromosome 1. The search for other risk factors generally has been unrewarding, no consistent evidence shows that infection, chemicals, or diet are involved in its cause. Furthermore, despite the strong effect of sex on the disease, no clear epidemiological evidence exists that reproductive or hormonal factors are important.

Epidemiology of systemic lupus erythematosus	
Prevalence	0.03%
Sex ratio	9:1 (women:men)

Scleroderma

In population surveys, the prevalence of scleroderma varies between 4 and 290 per million. Its annual incidence seems to be more constant at around 10 per million and is highest in the fifth and sixth decades. The woman:man excess is 3:1-8:1. Scleroderma is more common in black people than white people in the United States, but the condition is rare in African countries. A genetic contribution to the disease is suggested by isolated reports of familial clustering. Weak associations have been shown with human leucocyte antigen, including human leucocyte antigen-DR3 and human leucocyte antigen-DR5, and seem stronger in subgroups defined by certain antibodies.

An environmental association is suggested by the observation that two scleroderma-like syndromes—the toxic oil syndrome and the eosinophilia-myalgia syndrome—have a definite environmental basis. A higher risk of scleroderma is reported among miners exposed to silica dust, and case reports exist of the disease in patients exposed to organic solvents and drugs including bleomycin and carbidopa. Recent interest, generated initially by case reports, has been in a possible association between scleroderma and exposure to silicone as a result of augmentation mammoplasty. This possible association has since failed to be confirmed in large, well designed cohort studies. All studies that investigate risk factors for scleroderma are limited by problems of definition of disease and past exposure and by the rarity of the disease itself. Scleroderma is associated with an increased mortality risk with a standardised mortality ratio of about 5 for all forms of the disease combined. The risk is greatest in those in whom the lung, kidney, and heart are affected. Pulmonary hypertension is an under-recognised and fatal complication, particularly of limited scleroderma.

Epidemiology of scleroderma	
Prevalence	4-290 per million
Annual incidence	10 per million
Increased mortality risk	Standardised mortality ratio of 5

Possible environmental causes for scleroderma

- Silica dust
- Organic solvents
- Drugs
  - Bleomycin
  - Carbidopa

Raynaud's phenomenon

Estimates of the prevalence of Raynaud's phenomenon vary between 2% and 17%. Most series report a woman to man excess of around 2 : 1. The wide variation in prevalence between studies is accounted for partly by differences in disease definition and by climatic variation in the countries where they were conducted. The prevalence of Raynaud's phenomenon, however, has also been shown to vary within the same geographical region among different racial groups. A genetic predisposition exists: twin studies indicate a heritability of about 50%. Case control studies show that the risk of disease in relatives of affected individuals is increased fivefold compared with that in the general population.

Raynaud's phenomenon occurs in the context of several diseases (including autoimmune rheumatic diseases and hypothyroidism) and after specific occupational exposures (including use of vibrating tools). The risk of developing rheumatic disease in those with initially isolated Raynaud's phenomenon has been estimated recently at three per 100 patients, with features of rheumatic disease developing on average 10 years after the onset of Raynaud's. Risk factors for progression to autoimmune disease include the presence of antinuclear antibodies.

Vasculitides

Population data on vasculitides other than temporal arteritis are sparse because of their rarity. The data are also difficult to assess because of the different schemes used for classification. The prevalence of Behçet's syndrome shows marked geographical variation. It is most common in the "silk route" countries of the Mediterranean (the prevalence of the syndrome in Turkey has been reported to be as high as 3 per 1000), the Middle East, Asia, China, and Japan. An association with human leucocyte antigen-B51 has been reported in those with severe disease. Polyarteritis nodosa (here including classical polyarteritis and microscopic polyangiitis) has an annual incidence in adult populations of approximately five per million and a prevalence of five per 100 000. The frequency of disease is similar in men and women. Some evidence suggests that its frequency has been increasing in recent years. Wegener's granulomatosis also has a prevalence of around five per 100 000 in white people, with an equal frequency in men and women. The disease shows wide geographical and seasonal variation, which may implicate an environmental trigger. Other vasculitides, including hypersensitivity vasculitis, Churg-Strauss syndrome, and Henoch–Schönlein purpura, each have a reported prevalence of three per 100 000 or less in the adult population.

Low back pain

About 40% of adults will have complained of an episode of back pain in the last year and 80% have had back pain at some point in their lives. Many studies report a peak in prevalence around the age of 60 years. A slight female excess is seen, which is more apparent among those who report chronic pain. Continuous pain accounts for about one quarter of the total prevalence.

Reported lower back pain is related to the extent of degenerative disease documented on magnetic resonance images. An individual's susceptibility to disc degeneration documented by magnetic resonance imaging and their tendency to report back pain has an important genetic basis. Environmental risk factors and associations with occupations have been reported. Low work satisfaction has been shown to predict back pain up to a decade later. Depression, multiple somatic symptoms, and poor health status are associated with

---

Epidemiology of Raynaud's phenomenon

- Prevalence: up to 15%
- Strong familial clustering for isolated disease
- Antinuclear antibodies predict subsequent development of autoimmune disease in a minority of patients

---

Risk factors and associations with Raynaud's phenomenon

Proposed risk factors for occurrence of the isolated disease
- Alcohol use
- High diastolic blood pressure
- Low body mass index

Reported associations
- Migraine
- Angina

Epidemiology of vasculitides

- Overall prevalence about 40 per 100 000 in adult populations in northern Europe
- Significant disease specific variations in occurrence reflect a variety of genetic and environmental triggers

---

Environmental risk factors and occupational associations implicated in pain reporting

Environmental risk factors
- Body height
- Recent pregnancy
- Use of oral contraceptives
- Cigarette smoking

Occupational associations
- Heavy lifting
- Whole body vibration

119

back pain, although whether these are causes or consequences is less clear. Low social class and poor educational achievement are also associated.

Regional pain, fibromyalgia, and chronic widespread pain

Over 80% of the population will consult with a general practitioner for regional or generalised pain and a significant number of these will be disabled by it. As with low back pain, mechanical, psychological, and social factors are implicated. The contribution of genetic factors is increasingly recognised.

Around one fifth of those who report musculoskeletal pain report symptoms that are widespread and chronic. Criteria have been developed to classify these patients as having the syndromes of chronic widespread pain and fibromyalgia—the latter being defined most often through the presence of tender points. Considerable overlap is seen in the patterns of occurrence and risk factors for widespread pain, fibromyalgia, and regional pain, which suggests that they may form part of the same spectrum of pain experience.

Rheumatology in the tropics

Data on rheumatic diseases in tropical countries have been difficult to collect systematically and still are emerging. The burden of musculoskeletal disease in these areas, however, should not be underestimated. The economic impact of disease inevitably is greater in societies with a high dependence on manual work, and outcomes are worse where healthcare provision is limited.

As in the west, knee osteoarthritis dominates as a cause of disability in the tropics. Osteoporosis is of increasing importance in Asia and the Far East as their populations age. As might be expected, septic arthritis and other arthropathies that result from infections by parasites, *Mycobacteria*, *Brucella*, fungi, and viruses are represented more commonly. Cases of rheumatic fever and rheumatic heart disease are now almost exclusively confined to the tropics. Reactive arthritis appears to be more common (and increasingly so in Africa in relation to the spread of HIV), although many reported cases may represent an uncharacterised acute infection. The prevalence of ankylosing spondylitis reflects the population frequency of human leucocyte antigen-B27: it is relatively rare in Africa but more common in Papua New Guinea. Gout is reported to be rare in African populations. Rheumatoid arthritis and systemic lupus erythematosus are reported to be less severe, although the extent to which this reflects differences in genetic susceptibility or the effects of selection and survival is to be established.

Prevalence of regional and general pain

Condition	Prevalence (%)
Elbow and forearm pain	9-12
Carpal tunnel syndrome	5
Chronic widespread pain	10
Fibromyalgia	2

Approximate number of expected patients with musculoskeletal disease in an average general practice list of 2000 patients aged 18-90 years

	Women	Men	Total
Chronic back pain	70	70	140
Osteoarthritis	50	30	80
Osteoporosis	50	15	65
Soft tissue rheumatism	10	9	19
Rheumatoid arthritis	10	3	13
Polymyalgia rheumatica	8	2	10
Ankylosing spondylitis	1	6	7
Systemic lupus erythematosus	1	0	1

Further reading

- Silman AJ, Hochberg MC. *Epidemiology of the rheumatic diseases*. Oxford: Oxford University Press, 2001

The data used in the graph on prevalence are taken from Office for National Statistics. *Living in Britain*. London: Stationery Office, 2000. The data used in the figure on consultation rates are taken from Office for National Statistics. *Morbidity statistics from general practice—fourth national study 1991–92*. London: Stationery Office, 2000

Index

Page numbers in **bold** type refer to figures; those in *italic* refer to boxed material.

ACE inhibitors   *85*, *90*, 91
acetabular labrum tear   21, **21**
Achilles tendon affections   *26*, 27, **27**, 28, 62, 72
acne remedies   94
acute gouty arthritis   39, 40
acute phase response   104, *104*
adalimumab   *59*
adhesive capsulitis   12, *12*
alcohol
   gout   41, 43, *43*, *117*
   osteoporosis   46, *46*, 48
   Raynaud's phenomenon   *119*
alkaline phosphatase   *104*, 105, *105*
allopurinol   43, *43*
alopecia   81, **81**
anaemia   *103*, 104
   rheumatoid arthritis   53, *53*, 54
   systemic lupus erythematosus   81, *81*
anakinra   *59*
analgesics *see* pain relief
ankles, swelling   69
ankylosing spondylitis   61, *61*, 64, **64**, 65, *66*
   back pain   16, 17
   epidemiology   116, *116*
   feet   28, **28**
   genetic factors   109
   hips   20
   neck immobility   11
annular tears   18
antibiotics, sexually-acquired arthritis   66–7
antidepressants, in fibromyalgia   32
anti-DNA antibodies   107
antifilaggrin antibodies   108
antimalarials *see* hydroxychloroquine
antineutrophil cytoplasmic antibodies   108
antinuclear antibodies   *92*, 93, 94, 107–9, *107*
antiphospholipid antibodies   108, *108*
antiphospholipid antibody syndrome   80, 83–6, 101
anti-tumour necrosis factor α   66, 72, 73, *73*
   see also etanercept; infliximab
apatite associated destructive osteoarthritis   36
arm pain   *8*, 10–14
aseptic necrosis   25, 78
atrial myxoma   101
autoantibodies   106–7, *107*
   Raynaud's phenomenon   87
   scleroderma   89, *89*, **89**
autoimmune diseases   8, 80, 92
   Raynaud's phenomenon in   87
   see also systemic lupus erythematosus
autoimmunity, organ-specific   92
autologous stem cell bone marrow
         transplantation   74
avascular necrosis, femoral head   20, *20*, **20**
azathioprine   *59*, 66, 78, *79*, 82
   systemic lupus erythematosus   85, *85*

back pain *see* low back pain
bacterial infection   65, 72
   elbow pain   14
   hip pain   19

reactive arthritis   61–2, *69*
vasculitides   100, **100**
"Baker's cysts"   22, 69
Behçet's syndrome   *94*, 118
biochemical investigations   105–6
biological agents   59, 72
bisphosphonates   *48*
"boggy" swellings   4, 53
bone biochemistry   *104*, 105–6, *105*
bone densitometry   47, *47*, **47**
bone mineral density   45–9
botulinum toxin therapy   9
Bouchard's nodes   7, **7**, 36
brachial neuritis   13
bursitis
   elbow   14, *14*, **14**
   hip   20–1
   knee   22
   olecranon   14, *14*, **14**
   plantar region   **25**, **26**
   shoulder   *12*
   trochanteric   20–1
buttock pain   17, 18, 20, 61, 62

calcaneal diseases   26, *26*
calcifying tendinitis   12
calcium, dietary supplementation   *48*
calcium channel blockers   *85*, *90*
calcium pyrophosphate arthritis   4, 8, 36, 39
capsaicin therapy   38
cardiovascular symtoms   82
   rheumatoid arthritis   *53*
   vasculitis   98, 99, 101
carpal tunnel   4
carpal tunnel syndrome   4, 5, **5**
catastrophic antiphospholipid syndrome   83–4
cauda equina syndrome   16–17
cervical spine   11, 51, **51**, 69
   see also vertebrae
cheiroarthropathy   *4*, 8, **8**
children   *72*
   abuse of   69, 71
   foot pain   23
   hip pain   19, *19*
   juvenile idiopathic arthritis   68–74
   knee pain   21
cholesterol embolism   101, **101**
chondrocalcinosis   8, **8**, **36**
chronic gouty arthritis   39, **39**
chronic upper-limb pain syndrome   *8*, 9
Churg-Strauss syndrome   98, *98*, 99, *119*
coagulation abnormalities   104, 108, *108*
complement   108–9, *109*
complementary medicine   32, 59
congenital dislocation of the hip   19, **19**
connective tissue diseases
   diagnosis   92–7
   see also antiphospholipid antibody syndrome; Raynaud's
         phenomenon; scleroderma; systemic lupus erythematosus
corticosteroids *see* steroids
cranial arteritis   **75**

Index

C reactive protein 104, *104*
"CREST" syndrome 88–9, *89*
cryoglobulinaemia *98*, 99, **99**
crystal associated osteoarthritis 36, 38
cubital tunnel syndrome *4, 7*
cutaneous scleroderma *87*, 88
cyclooxygenase II selective agents 56–7, *56*, 66
cyclophosphamide *59*, 74, 79
  systemic lupus erythematosus 85, *85*
  toxicity 102
  vasculitides 101–2
cyclosporin *59*, 79, *79*, 85, *85*
cytotoxic drugs 85, *85*

dactylitis 8, 28, **28**, **62**
depression 2, 10, 76, 81
  back pain 119
  fibromyalgia 30–2
De Quervain's tenosynovitis *4, 6*, **6**
dermatomyositis 92, *94*, 95, **95**
  juvenile 70, **70**
diabetes
  frozen shoulder 12
  stiff hand *4, 8*
diet, arthritis and 60, *60*
discs, prolapsed *15*, 16, **16**
disease-modifying antirheumatic drugs 58, *58–60*, 66
diuretics, gout induced by 40
D-penicillamine *59*
drug-induced lupus 92, 94–5
drug therapy
  bone mass increase 48, *48*
  giant cell arteritis 78
  gout 42
  juvenile idiopathic arthritis 72
  osteoarthritis 37–8, *38*
  polymyalgia rheumatica 78
  Raynaud's phenomenon 85, *90*
  rheumatoid arthritis 56–9
  spondyloarthropathy 66
  systemic lupus erythematosus *84*, 85–6
  thrombosis in antiphospholipid antibody syndrome 86
  vasculitides 101–2
Dupuytren's contracture *4, 7*, **7**, *8*

elbows
  pain 10, 13–14, *13*, *51*, 52
  skin changes 88
enteropathic arthritis *66*
enthesitis 62, 71–2, *71*
environmental disease 117
epicondylitis **13**, 13–14, *13*
erythrocyte sedimentation rate 104, *104*
etanercept *59*, 66, 73, *73*
evidence-based care 3, 111
exercise 32, *48*
extensor tenosynovitis *4, 6*
eyes
  chronic anterior uveitis 63
    childhood 71, 72
  conjunctivitis *62*, 63, **63**
  scleritis 52, **52**
  vision loss 76, 78, *78*
  see also Sjögren's syndrome

face *see* mouth; photosensitivity
facet arthrosis/syndrome 17
fatigue 52, *52*, 75, 76, 81, *88*, 92, 94, 95
feet 23–9
  enthesitis related arthritis 72
  gout **39**
  juvenile idiopathic arthritis 69
  rheumatoid arthritis *51*, 52

spondyloarthropathy **62**, 63, **63**
  see also ankles; heels; toes
Felty's syndrome *103*
fibromyalgia 30–2, *94*, 96, 120
  childhood 69, 71
fingers 4–8
  connective tissue disease **93**, *95*
  cutaneous scleroderma 88, **88**
  ischaemic damage *95*, **95**
  Raynaud's phenomenon 87, **87**
  tendon problems 5–6
  see also nails
first carpometacarpal osteoarthritis *4*, 6, 7
flexor tendonosis *4, 6*
flexor tenosynovitis *4*, 5, **5**, 6, 8, **8**
forearm pain 13–14
Freiberg's infraction (osteochondritis) 25
frozen shoulder 12, *12*

ganglion *4, 8*
gastrointestinal infection, Reiter's syndrome 116
gastrointestinal symptoms 82, 91, *98*, 99
  NSAID toxicity 57, *57*
general practitioners 111, *111*
genetic factors
  osteoporosis 47, *47*
  rheumatic disease 109, 114–20
genitourinary infection, Reiter's syndrome 116
genitourinary system, spondyloarthropathy 63,
  66–7
giant cell arteritis 75–9, 117–18
glenohumoral joint arthritides 12–13
glenoid labrum injuries 13
glucosamine 38
gold therapy *58*
Gottron's papules 70, **70**
gout 22, 39–43, 117, *117*

haematological changes
  antiphospholipid antibody syndrome 83
  rheumatoid arthritis 53
  systemic lupus erythematosus 81
haematological investigations 103–5
hands 4–9
  connective tissue disease **95**
  osteoarthritis 36, **36**
  photosensitivity 96
  psoriasis 63, **63**, **65**
  rheumatoid arthritis **50**, 51, *51*, 52, **55**
  synovitis, juvenile idiopathic arthritis 69
Heberden's nodes 7, **7**, 36
heels, painful 26–7
Henoch-Schönlein purpura 70, *98*, 99, 119
hips 19–21
  osteoarthritis **34**, *35*, 36, **36**, 37, 115
  osteoporotic fractures 20, **20**, 115–16, *115*
  rheumatoid arthritis *51*, 52
HIV infection 16, 117
hormone replacement therapy *48*
hydroxychloroquine *58*, 74, 79
  systemic lupus erythematosus 82, 83, 85, *85*
hyperalgesia, in fibromyalgia 30–1
hypermobility, and joint pain 69, *69*
hyperuricaemia 39, 40–3
hypogonadism, in osteoporosis 46, *46*, 47

ilio-psoas tendons, snapping 21
imaging
  juvenile idiopathic arthritis *71*
  lumbar spine 16
  neck or shoulder pain 11
  rheumatoid arthritis 54–5
  spondyloarthropathy 64, **64**

immunoglobulins 108
immunological investigations 106
industrial disease, scleroderma 118
infections 75, *94*, 109
infective arthritis 8
infective endocarditis 100–1, **101**
inflammatory arthritis 1, 2, *4*, 7–8
   childhood 69–70, 72
   foot 25
   neck pain 11
   see also rheumatoid arthritis; spondyloarthropathies
inflammatory bowel disease 61, *61*, 62, 63, 72
infliximab *59*, 66, 73, *73*
intervertebral discs, prolapsed *15*, 16, **16**
intra-articular steroids *see* steroids, intra-articular
"irritable hip" 19

Janeway lesions 100–1, **101**
Jessner's benign lymphocytic infiltration *94*, 96, **96**
joint aspiration, spondyloarthropathy 64
joints
   hypermobility 69, *69*
   inflamed *72*
   swelling 11, 21, 62, **62**, 68–9
      see also juvenile idiopathic arthritis; spondyloarthropathy
   see also under specific joints
juvenile chronic arthritis *see* juvenile idiopathic arthritis
juvenile dermatomyositis 70, **70**
juvenile idiopathic arthritis 19, 23, 68–74

Kawasaki disease 70, **70**, 98, *98*
keyboard use *8*, 8
Kienboeck disease *4*, 9
knees 21–2
   osteoarthritis *35*, 36, 37, 115
   rheumatoid arthritis *51*, 52
   skin changes 88
   swelling 68–9, **68**

laboratory findings 103–9
   antiphospholipid antibody syndrome *83*, 84
   juvenile idiopathic arthritis *71*
   polymyalgia rheumatica 77–8
   rheumatoid arthritis 54, 104–7, *104, 106, 107*
   spondyloarthropathy 63–4, *63*
   systemic lupus erythematosus 84, 104–7, *104, 106, 107*
   vasculitides 100
lead exposure *42*, 117, *117*
leflunomide *58*
leg pain 16–17
ligament injuries, knee 21, 22
limited joint mobility syndrome 8
livedo reticularis 100, **100**, 101
liver function tests *104*, 105, *105*
low back pain 15–18, 119–20
   red flag symptoms *17*
   risk factors 118–19
lumbar root lesions *15*, **15**, 16
lumbar spine **15**, 16, **17**
   imaging 16
lungs
   fibrosis 90, *90*
   pulmonary hypertension 82, 89, **89**, 90
   rheumatoid arthritis 53
   scleroderma 89, **89**, 90
   vasculitis *98*, 99
lupus
   drug induced *92*, 94–5
   see also systemic lupus erythematosus
lupus anticoagulant test *108*

malaise 52, *52*, 70, 81, 92
malignancy 10, 15, 16, 20, 70, *70*, 72

manual work 8, 10, *13*
meniscal tear, knee 21, **21**, 22
menopausal osteoarthritis 36, **36**
metatarsalgia 23–4
methotrexate *58*, 66, 79, *79*, 85, *85*
   in childhood 72, 73, *73*
microbiology 109
microscopic polyangiitis 98, *98*, 99
minocycline 94
miscarriage recurrence 83, *83*, 86
morning pain 5
morning stiffness 16, *17*, 62, 81
Morton's neuroma 23–4
mouth
   microstomia **88**
   stiffness 69
   ulcers *80*, 81
   see also Sjögren's syndrome
mucocutaneous lymph node syndrome 70,
   70, 98, *98*
"Mulder's click" 23
muscle "knots" 11
muscular weakness 70
musculoskeletal pain 120
musical instrument, injury 9
mycophenolate mofetil 85, *85*
myofascial pain 11

nailfold disorders 87, *95*, 99
nails, psoriatic 63, **63**, **65**
neck pain 10–14
necrotising vasculitides 98–9, 100
neonatal lupus syndrome 82
neoplasia 70, *70*
nerve entrapment
   elbow 7, 14
   foot 23–4
nerve root lesions, low back pain
   15, **15**, 16
neuritis, brachial plexus 13
neurological features
   neck pain 11
   rheumatoid arthritis 53
   systemic lupus erythematosus 81–2
nocturnal pain 10–11, *17*, 70, *70*
nodal osteoarthritis *4*, 7, **7**, 36, **36**
nodules, rheumatoid 52, **52**
non-steroidal anti-inflammatory drugs 56–7, *56, 57*,
   66, 78, 85
   in childhood 72, 73
numbness 5
nurse specialists 1, 112, *112*

occupational disorders 114, *119*, 120
occupational therapists 112, *112*
oesophageal symptoms *88*, 90, 91
oestrogen deficiency 46, *46*, 48
olecranon bursitis 14, *14*, **14**
oligoarthritis, childhood 71, *71*
Osgood-Schlatter disease 21, 26
osteoarthritis 34–8, 110–11, 115
   foot 27, **27**
   hand and wrist *4*, 7, **7**
   hip 20, **20**
   knee 22, **22**
   nodal 8, **8**
   risk factors *115*
osteochondritis dessicans 22
osteochondritis (Freiberg's infraction) 25
osteomyelitis 70
osteonecrosis *4*, 8
osteoporosis 20, 24, 45–9, 53, 115–16
overlap syndromes 93, *93*, 95

Index

Paget's disease 20, 105, *105*, 106
pain relief
  fibromyalgia 32
  osteoarthritis 37
  osteoporosis 48
  rheumatoid arthritis 56–7, *56*, *57*
pain syndromes, childhood 70–1, *70*
palindromic rheumatism 51
patella subluxation 21
patient care, team approach 1–3, 110–12
Perthes disease 19
Phalen's test 5
photosensitivity 80, 82, *84*, 85, *94*, 95–6
physiotherapy 3, 56, *56*, 65, 111, *111*, 112
pins and needles 5, 7
plantar disorders 25–6, **25**, 26, **29**, **64**
platelet abnormalities 103
podiatry 23, 28–9, 112
policeman's heel 26
polyarteritis nodosa 98, *98*, **99**, **100**, 101, 119
polymorphous light eruption *94*, 96, **96**
polymyalgia rheumatica 75–9, *76*, 117–18
polymyositis *92*
popliteal cysts 22
pregnancy
  antiphospholipid antibody syndrome 83, *83*
  rheumatoid arthritis *50*, 57
  systemic lupus erythematosus 82, *82*, 84, *84*, 85
premature onset osteoarthritis 36, *36*
pseudogout *4*, 8, 22, 39
psoriatic arthritis 7, 28, **28**, 61, *61*, 63, **63**, 64, **64**, 65, *65*
  epidemiology 116–17, *116*
  risk factors *117*
psoriatic juvenile idiopathic arthritis 71
psychosocial factors, chronicity and 2, *2*
pulmonary symptoms *see* lungs

radiculopathies 14
rashes
  childhood inflammatory arthritis **69**, 70
  connective tissue diseases *93*, *94*, 95–6, **97**
  systemic lupus erythematosus *80*, 81, **81**, *84*, 85
  vasculitides and 98–102
Raynaud's phenomenon *4*, 8, 85, *85*, 87–91
  connective tissue diseases *93*, 94, 95
  epidemiology 118, *118*
  risk factors *118*
reactive arthritis 61, *61*, 63, **63**, 65, *65*
  childhood 69, *69*, 72
referred pain
  from hip 20, 21
  to spine 15, 16
regional pain syndromes, "red flags" 2
Reiter's syndrome 22, **28**, 116, *116*
renal disease 81
  drug induced lupus 94–5
  function tests *104*, 105, *105*
  NSAIDS and 56–7, *57*
  rheumatoid arthritis 52, *52*, **52**
  scleroderma renal crisis 91
  systemic lupus erythematosus 80
  urate stones 42
  vasculitis 98, 99
repetitive use 5, *6*, 14
respiratory symptoms *98*
rheumatic diseases
  care provision 1–3, 110–12
  chronicity prediction 2, *2*
  epidemiology 114–20
rheumatoid arthritis 7–8, *7*, 50–5
  care standards 110–11
  differential diagnosis 94, *94*, 95
  epidemiology 114–15

feet 24, **24**, 27, **27**, **29**
genetic factors 109
gout and 40
hip 20
juvenile form 72
knee 22
laboratory findings 104–7, *104*, *106*, *107*
neck pain 11
risk/protective factors *115*
Sjögren's syndrome 82–3
treatment 56–60
rheumatoid factors 106, *106*
rheumatology care 1–3, 110–12
rosacea *94*, 96, **96**
rotator cuff lesions 11–12, *12*

sacroiliac pain 18, *18*, **18**
sacroiliitis 62, 64, **64**
"sausage" digits 8, 28, **28**, *62*
scalp tenderness 76
scaphoid bone fracture *4*, 8–9
scapulothoracic pain *13*
sciatica 16
scleroderma 87–91, 118, *118*
seborrhoeic dermatitis *94*, 96
selective oestrogen receptor modulators *48*
self-help 3, 31–2, 37, *37*
self-management 111, 112
septic arthritis 21–2, **22**, 39, 42, 72
  childhood 19, 69–70, *72*
  hip 20
seronegative arthritis 7
Sever's disease 26
shoulders 10–14, 51, *51*, 75, 76
Sjögren's syndrome 52, *52*, 80, 82–3, 85, *92*, 95, 96
skin changes 8, 87–91, *98*
  see also rashes
"skip" phenomenon 77, *77*
sleep disturbance 30, *31*, 32, 71
slipped upper femoral epiphysis 19
smoking 46, *46*, *48*, 115–16, *115*
soft tissue pad, metatarsal 24–5
sphincter disturbance 17
spine
  spinal stenosis 16
  spondyloarthropathies 17, 28, 61–7
    see also ankylosing spondylitis;
      enteropathic arthritis; psoriatic arthritis;
      reactive arthritis
  spondylolysis/spondylolisthesis 17–18
  see also cervical spine; low back pain; vertebrae
sports-related injuries 17–18, 21, 24, 25, 35
steroids
  adverse events 78, 82
  childhood 73, *73*
  infection and 96–7
  intra-articular 38, 73, *73*
    contra-indications 3, 21
    technique (hand/wrist) 3, 4–5, **5**, 6, **6**
  polymyalgia rheumatica/giant cell
    arteritis 78
  pregnancy 82
  rheumatoid arthritis 57–8, *57*
  spondyloarthropathy 66
  systemic lupus erythematosus 85
  vasculitides 101–2
steroid sparing agents 79, *79*, 85, *85*
Still's disease *see* juvenile idiopathic arthritis
straight leg raise test **16**
stress fractures 17–18, *24*
student's elbow 14, *14*, **14**
subacromial impingement **10**, 12
sulfasalazine *58*, 66, 72, 73, *73*, 94

surgery
  osteoarthritis   38
  Raynaud's phenomenon   *90*
  rheumatoid arthritis   56, *56*
  spondyloarthropathy   65
synovitis   4, 24
  juvenile idiopathic arthritis   68–9
  polymyalgia rheumatica   77
  spondyloarthropathy   61
systemic arthritis, childhood   72, *72*
systemic lupus erythematosus   80–3, 84–6, 118
  antibodies in   *92*, 93
  childhood   70
  fibromyalgia and   96
  infection and   96–7
  laboratory findings   104–7, *104, 106, 107*
systemic sclerosis   88–9, *92, 94*, 95, **96**

Takayasu's arterits   98, *98*
tarsal coalition   23, **25**
temporal arteritis   75
temporomandibular synovitis   69
tendon disorders
  hand and wrist   5–6
  hip   21
  shoulder   12, *12*, 13, 14
thoracic outlet syndrome   13
thrombocytopenia   103, *103*
thrombosis   83–4, *83*, 84
thumb, functional anatomy   4
thyroid disease, frozen shoulder   12
Tinel's sign   5, 7
tingling   5
toes   24, **24**, 25, **25**, 27–8, **27**, *28*, **28**, **62**
  gout   39, **39**
tophaceous gout   40
transient synovitis   19
trauma
  foot   23
  hand and wrist   4, 8–9
  knee   21

osteoarthritis   35
shoulder injuries   13
synovitis   24
whiplash injury   11
trigger finger/thumb   *4*, 6, **6**
trochanteric bursitis   20–1
tropics, rheumatology in   120
tumour necrosis factor[-alpha] blockade   79, *79*

undifferentiated connective tissue disease   93–4, *93*, **93**
upper arm pain   *8*, 10–14
urate metabolism   40–3

vascular disease   52, *52*, 82, *82*
  see also Raynaud's phenomenon
vasculitides   98–102, 119, *119*
  childhood   70
  differential diagnosis   *94*, 100
  systemic   75–9
vasodilators   *90*
vertebrae
  in ankylosing spondylitis   64, **64**
  disc prolapse   *15*, 16, **16**
  fractures   47, **47**, 78, 115
  see also cervical spine; low back pain
vibration white finger   8, 87, *87*, 119
viral infection
  hip pain   19
  reactive arthritis   *69*
  shoulder pain   13

Wegener's granulomatosis   98, *98*, **98**, **99**, 101, 119
weight loss   70, 75, 76, *76*, 81, *88*, 94
Whipple's disease   62, **62**, 65
white blood cell abnormalities   104
work-related disorders
  upper-limb pain   4, 8, *8*, 9
  see also manual work
wrist   4–9, 51, *51*, 52, 69
writer's cramp   *4*, 9

The complete ABC series

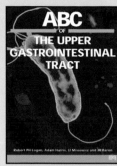

ABC of AIDS
ABC of Alcohol
ABC of Allergies
ABC of Antenatal Care
ABC of Antithrombotic Therapy
ABC of Asthma
ABC of Arterial and Venous Disease
ABC of Arterial and Venous Disease, CD ROM
ABC of Brain Stem Death
ABC of Breast Diseases
ABC of Child Abuse
ABC of Clinical Electrocardiography
ABC of Clinical Genetics
ABC of Clinical Haematology
ABC of Colorectal Cancer
ABC of Colorectal Diseases
ABC of Complementary Medicine
ABC of Dermatology (includes CD ROM)
ABC of Diabetes
ABC of Emergency Radiology
ABC of Eyes (includes CD ROM)
ABC of the First Year
ABC of Heart Failure
ABC of Hypertension
ABC of Intensive Care
ABC of Interventional Cardiology
ABC of Labour Care
ABC of Learning and Teaching in Medicine
ABC of Liver, Pancreas and Gall Bladder
ABC of Major Trauma
ABC of Mental Health
ABC of Nutrition
ABC of Occupational and Environmental Medicine
ABC of One to Seven
ABC of Oral Health
ABC of Otolaryngology
ABC of Palliative Care
ABC of Psychological Medicine
ABC of Resuscitation
ABC of Rheumatology
ABC of Sexual Health
ABC of Sexually Transmitted Infections
ABC of Spinal Cord Injury
ABC of Sports Medicine
ABC of Subfertility
ABC of Transfusion
ABC of the Upper Gastrointestinal Tract
ABC of Urology

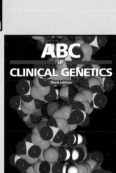

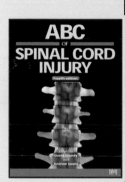

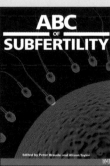

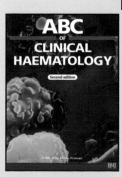

Titles are available from all good medical bookshops or visit:

www.abc.bmjbooks.com